Advance Praise for

The Estrogen Answer Book

"Ruth Jacobowitz has done it again! *The Estrogen Answer Book* is a well-researched, unbiased assessment of the treatments available for management of menopausal symptoms as well as preventive strategies to maintain health in the second half of our lives. I will recommend it not only for all of my patients entering midlife, but for my friends and family as well."
— Barbara Levy, M.D.
Clinical Assistant Professor of Obstetrics/Gynecology
Yale University School of Medicine

"As millions of women move into their menopausal years, the 'estrogen decision' becomes an issue of great importance. Ruth Jacobowitz's new book is a most valuable resource that will help women make this decision in an informed and educated manner."
—Susan M. Lark, M.D.
author of *The Estrogen Decision Self Help Book*

"*The Estrogen Answer Book* guides women through the maze of issues and questions regarding hormone replacement therapy and menopause. This is an extremely well written reference for women who are about to enter menopause, as well as those who are frustrated and confused by the myriad of treatment options. Ruth Jacobowitz has provided a valuable resource for the growing number of women experiencing menopause."
—R. Jeffrey Chang, M.D.
Director, D[...]y and Infertility
Departm[...]Medical Center

D0967768

The
Estrogen
Answer Book

150 Most-Asked Questions
About Hormone
Replacement Therapy

Ruth S. Jacobowitz

Little, Brown and Company

Boston New York Toronto London

First Edition

The ideas, suggestions and answers to questions in this book are not intended to substitute for the help and services of a trained professional. All matters regarding your health require medical consultation and supervision, and following any of the advice and procedures in this book should be done in conjunction with the services of a qualified health professional.

Library of Congress Cataloging-in-Publication Data
Jacobowitz, Ruth S.
     The estrogen answer book : 150 most-asked questions about hormone replacement therapy / Ruth S. Jacobowitz. — 1st ed.
          p. cm.
     Includes index.
     ISBN 0-316-45808-2
     1. Menopause — Hormone therapy — Miscellanea.   2. Estrogen — Therapeutic use — Miscellanea.   3. Middle-aged women — Health and hygiene — Miscellanea.   I. Title.
     RG129.H6J33   1998
     618.1'7506 — dc21   98-25178

10 9 8 7 6 5 4 3 2 1

MV-NY

Book design: Barbara Werden Design

Published simultaneously in Canada by
Little, Brown & Company (Canada) Limited
Printed in the United States of America

This book is dedicated to my daughters,
Jan, Jody, and Julie, and
to women everywhere, with
the hope that it will help them make
informed decisions about their health
and their health care, so they
can live longer and better lives

Contents

Part Four: Making the Decision

Foreword

ODAY the life span of a healthy woman is expected to last well into her eighties. In 1900 a woman's life expectancy rarely exceeded fifty years of age. A sixty-five-year-old woman in excellent health can expect 16.8 more years of active life. These statistics point out that today a woman lives more than half her life without the benefit of her own estrogen. The time from menarche to menopause, the time when she is making her own estrogen, is but a brief part of her total life span. It is therefore very important that every woman know the answers to the important questions about estrogen, and be able to make informed decisions on her reproductive health. Ruth Jacobowitz has written a powerful book that addresses the issues that should be of paramount importance to every woman and that are key to a woman's entire life.

Although estrogen is recognized as an important part of the risk factors in three of the most prevalent female cancers, not as much attention has been focused on the necessity for estrogen for the rest of the body. The definition of estrogen commonly identifies only the regulation and maintenance of female sexual development and reproductive function. But today we know that estrogen has a wider impact and plays a role in cardiovascular disease, osteoporosis (loss of bone density), urological function (incontinence), skin turgor, and perhaps even cognitive function (dementia).

Cardiovascular disease is the leading cause of death among women between the ages of fifty and seventy-five. This represents a quarter of a million deaths each year.

Osteoporosis is a "silent killer"; 1.5 million fractures each year can be directly associated with postmenopausal osteoporosis. An older woman's risk of a hip fracture is equal to her risk for breast, uterine, and ovarian cancer combined.

Urinary incontinence affects approximately thirteen million Americans in community and institutional settings, 85 percent of whom are women. The pelvic floor supporting the bladder and urethra is anatomically vulnerable to estrogen deprivation. Estrogen is important to a woman's total well-being.

Future research and clinical trials will enhance our ability to make "designer choices." Targeted estrogen therapy replacement, unique receptor therapy, and attention to individual risk factors — for example, genetic and clotting factors — will bring more safety to hormone replacement. Selective estrogen receptor modulators (SERMs) are the beginning of a new era in identifying unique ways to isolate the good estrogen effects from the bad. Long-term research will be needed to ensure the risk-to-benefit advantages.

The consumer must also be part of the decision process. Many of the decisions must be made in adolescence, when patterns of good nutrition, exercise, and lifestyle are set. These years are critical for laying down sufficient bone to protect the older woman. The battle of the Law of Inertia must be fought each year. Every American adult should accumulate thirty minutes or more of moderate intensity exercise on most, if not all, days of the week. Today only 22 percent of Americans are currently active at this level. Lack of regular exercise contributes to as many as 250,000 deaths per year in the United States.

Women approaching menopause or already experiencing some of the effects should make every effort to become knowledgeable consumers. Ruth Jacobowitz has presented us with a convenient way to access a wide range of information gathered from a large assortment of authoritative resources. The question-

and-answer format is well suited to those of us who need a quick bit of information, and an in-depth read will provide a solid basis for making informed decisions.

Jean L. Fourcroy, M.D., Ph.D.
Past president, American Medical Women's Association
Past president, National Council on Women's Health
Board-certified urologist

Acknowledgments

THERE is no way that I could have begun, yet alone completed, this book without the help of many people. First of all I want to thank the thousands of women who have filled out my questionnaires, generously sharing with me their decisions about estrogen, along with their questions and concerns. There is no way a work such as this — consumer-oriented because it is consumer-driven — could have direction and meaning without their valuable input.

I want to thank all the professionals with whom I have worked over the years who have generously shared information with me and helped me to become a women's health advocate, knowing as they do the challenges awaiting individuals championing the cause of midlife women's health. I interviewed so many people for this book that any attempt to mention them all by name would be folly, for I would surely leave someone out. I am grateful to all of you who toil diligently, trying to sort out for your patients and for women everywhere what is right and good for them and what will enhance the quality of their lives and promote their longevity.

My editor, Jennifer Josephy, conceived of the idea of an estrogen book and agreed that we would publish not another menopause book but truly a book about estrogen. I must thank Jennifer for her support. I also want to thank Peter Sawyer, my agent, who put Jennifer and me together, enabling us to produce this book.

The unquestioning encouragement provided by my loving family has helped me through the writing of five books and has supported my speaking at seminars all over the world. My husband, Paul, and I are blessed with three wonderful daughters and three equally wonderful sons-in-law, who have given us eight fabulous grandchildren. I want to thank Jan Jacobowitz and Alvin Lodish for Jeffrey and Ryan; Jody and David Austin for Claire, Jake, and Lili; and Julie and Lowell Potiker for Michael, Cara, and Danielle. My undying love goes out to all of them each day.

The rest of the family pitches in, too, excusing my absences and letting me know that they are proud of me, which helps immeasurably when my energy slips and my direction falters. So, thanks to my sisters and my brothers-in-law, Harriet and Bud Lewis and Susan and Leonard Rosenberg, and to Paul's brother and my sister-in-law, Rifkie and Bill Jacobowitz. It takes a family to raise and nurture one another and to support individual efforts.

There are a few other people whom I must thank, who kept me on track: Denise Keeter, who taught me how to use my new computer and word processing program and came quickly to unscramble my computer mess-ups; Deanne Siegal, M.S., R.D., whose assistance was invaluable in the preparation of the calcium counter; and Eva Grausz, who came aboard at the end to compile and prepare some of the appendix materials. More thanks and hugs go to Kristen Lee, my acupuncturist, and Mara Carrico, my yoga instructor, who kept me sound of mind and body while I wrote this book.

Finally, I must again thank the women everywhere who over these past years have never failed to strengthen my resolve to educate and empower women so that we can live better while we are living longer.

Ruth S. Jacobowitz

The **Estrogen** Answer Book

Introduction

BEGAN thinking about the contents of this book long before I thought about writing it. One difficult question had plagued me for a long time. In fact, from the first moment I was prescribed estrogen for my disconcerting and somewhat debilitating menopause symptoms, I wondered, "Should I take estrogen?"

My entry into menopause left me little choice. Let me explain. Back when I was in my forties, not so very long ago, menopause was still a taboo subject, kept under wraps and barely whispered about. And so I fell headlong into the worst experience of my life. Having suffered with heavy menstrual bleeding for more than a year, and with anemia and embarrassment my constant companions, I finally decided to have a hysterectomy. It was just another one of the 600,000 that are done in the United States each year, two-thirds of which are probably unnecessary. Mine was undoubtedly unnecessary as well, but I didn't know that then. I only knew it seemed like a good idea at the time. Besides, my ovaries were still intact, so I didn't have to worry about surgically induced menopause. Or so I thought.

Just a few years later, I began to suffer. In the midst of a meeting I would break out in a sticky sweat. At night I was unbearably hot and sweaty. Did I think of menopause? Absolutely not. I did, however, mention the sweating to my gynecologist, who suggested I might try vitamin E. It helped enormously, and so I remained dry and in the dark for a few more years. That's strange, you must be thinking. After all, I am a medical writer who for many years was a vice president of a large Cleveland teaching hospital, so you must be wondering why I didn't figure out that I was making an important transition. Well, I didn't. But then, we didn't talk about things like perimenopause back then.

My nerves were shot and my moods swung widely, and yet I kept believing it was the toil and turmoil of hospital administration that was destroying me. A good night's sleep was becoming a rare occurrence and my heartbeat felt electric. I didn't even realize that palpitations were a common menopausal symptom.

One night I awoke hot and sweaty with such wild palpitations that I thought I was having a heart attack. The next day I felt anxious, weepy, and sad, but I couldn't even summon up the emotion to cry. I was so badly frightened, I panicked.

That panic, coupled with anxiety, lasted for weeks, during which I suffered insomnia to such an extent that I don't remember sleeping at all. Late-night television didn't help, because when I tried to watch, the colors seemed to run together and the effort was unsettling. Reading, my favorite pastime, was not possible either. I simply could not concentrate. Decision making was impossible, and I found myself crying in the car and in supermarkets and department stores. What had happened to me?

Finally, when my husband and children could bear it no longer, they forced me to see a physician. Did I choose to go to my physician-partner, a gynecologist friend with whom I had been sharing the responsibility for my good health? No way. I sought out a new young doctor in town who wouldn't know me either professionally or socially, stupidly thinking that would keep what I believed was my nervous breakdown secret. After all, if you think you are losing your mind, you don't want to share what's left of it with your business associates and friends. That was my biggest mistake. This brash young doctor offered me Valium (you remember Valium, the Prozac of the '80s) and never even bothered to check my hormone levels.

That sent me back to my gynecologist in a hurry. He listened to me relate my symptoms, checked my follicle-stimulating hormone levels, and prescribed estrogen. Within the first week on estrogen all my symptoms began to diminish, and by the end of the second week they were gone for good. Could all my discomfort and fright have just been caused by the symptoms of menopause? At first I doubted it, but I began to educate myself about menopause and to learn why I had such a terrible introduction to what have turned out to be the best years of my life. No, menopause does not rise up one night and catch you in its power; it is a rather subtle process that unless brought on by surgery takes several years to present itself fully. That's why it is such a good idea to pay attention to your symptoms and learn what is changing in your body. No surprises for you then.

Even back then I was troubled about having to take an estrogen replacement medication to offset the severe symptoms I was plagued with from a perfectly normal transition. So even though it had solved my problems, I kept asking myself, "Should I be taking estrogen?"

At first the question simply nagged at me. Then it began to follow me around. After my first book was published, it was asked of me professionally and socially. During a meeting with a prospective client, someone who wanted me to write or lecture, the question would invariably come up in one way or another.

In social settings women would come up to me and say, "I've read your books on menopause, but I'm still not sure what I should do." They would offer a brief menopause history in hushed tones and finally whisper the question, "Should I take estrogen?"

I would have loved to offer a simple yes or no, but the answers to that question are many and varied and frequently complicated. Women are too busy for puzzling answers. We women have that wonderful habit of wanting to make a satisfactory decision and "get on with it!" With a question about estrogen, that's simply not possible. There are more questions to be asked. One question begets another. There are questions about a woman's family medical history and about her own, and there are as many answers as there are issues surrounding menopause and hormone replacement therapy. We have to read, we have to learn. The decision to begin hormone replacement therapy may well be the most challenging, complex, and confusing decision that a healthy menopausal woman may have to make. The benefits of estrogen cannot be denied: it reduces or eliminates symptoms; it slows or stops bone loss; and there is strong evidence that it protects against heart disease and other diseases as well. But there remains the other consideration, that perhaps long-term hormone replacement therapy increases the risk of breast cancer.

Beginning with younger women, still flirting with perimenopause and their early queries about what they should do when they get to menopause, continuing on to women at menopause, and beyond them to postmenopausal women of all ages, one question prevails: "Should I take estrogen?" The question is asked unabashedly now, noncombatively but directly. I reviewed my earlier works and knew that although in 1993 I responded to lots of questions in *150 Most-Asked Questions About Menopause,* there were still other questions, piqued by more recent research, to be answered about estrogen and about nonhormonal therapies.

In 1994 I wrote *150 Most-Asked Questions About Osteoporosis,* which focused on preventing that bone deteriorating, crippling, killing disease and discussed estrogen; but there still remained some estrogen questions, based on the availability of new products, begging for answers. There weren't any more answers. Not then. There are quite a few new solutions now. And while lecturing about menopause and osteoporosis, I realized that information was still needed about what happens to our sexuality with the advent of menopause, and where our partners are in all the hormonal dips and swings, so next came *150 Most-Asked Questions About Midlife Sex, Love, and Intimacy,* in 1995. The books in that trilogy kept me circling the country and other places in the world lecturing. The women I met and talked with while I toured raised even more questions about estrogen. No matter where I went or to whom I spoke, the key question remained the same: "Should *I* take estrogen?"

So I began again, circulating questionnaires, interviewing

women of all appropriate ages and stages of life, talking with many of their partners, and returning to the experts for sound advice.

This book was written to help women sort through all the available information about estrogen. When armed with good information, a woman can decide what she wants to do when it is time to make her own estrogen decision. This book is designed to enable you to understand how estrogen may pertain to you and your situation. Above all, while you are digesting the information, don't forget that, although menopause is universal, it is also unique. By that I mean that menopause is a transition each woman will experience, but how it will affect her will be quite different from how her female family members, neighbors, co-workers, and friends are affected. Not all symptoms affect all of us, nor do the ones we experience affect someone else to the same degree. A hot flash to you may be an annoyance; hot flashes to another woman may be experienced as a life-altering series of symptoms.

Some women whose mates like a well-chilled bedroom may even welcome night sweats; others begin the unabated thermostat wars with their mates. She's hot; he's cold. Blankets and quilts and tempers fly. I use the hot flash here to make my point because it is the most common of all the symptoms of menopause, affecting 75 to 85 percent of women. The flash is not fun. It may come upon you as an aura, and then hit you in the face, reddening it and making it wet with perspiration. Although some T-shirts and bumper stickers proclaim "It's not a hot flash, it's a power surge!" I disagree. I prefer the black T-shirt with the large white letters that someone sent me that reads "I'm out of estrogen and I've got a gun!" I truly can't view the hot flash as a power surge; I view it more as a temporary power outage, similar to when the air-conditioning system fails during a heat wave. You want it fixed quickly!

Imagine, for just a moment, the female executive presenting a complex proposal to a group of her peers, men in suits, with perhaps a very young attractive secretary sitting in at the meeting, in the boardroom of a large corporation. Her presentation is exquisite, and the questioning concerning her proposal begins. She's holding her own, answering question after question. She knows instinctively that she's fielding them well.

Suddenly, a hot flash begins. Perhaps the heightened stress of the presentation has brought it forth. She feels the heat beginning at her waist and slowly, inexorably, climbing up her body. Under her suit jacket, her silk blouse begins to stick to her skin. The flash keeps moving upward, and when it hits her smack in the face she takes her file folder and begins to fan herself. Around the board table, to a man, they are wondering, "Why is she so nervous? What does she know that we don't know? Can we trust this plan of hers?"

Far-fetched? Not at all. Women play out similar scenarios daily. Trade the boardroom for the classroom, or anywhere else there is a group of people, and the picture remains the same. Embarrassing? Of course, and none of us has really taken that giant step to where we can say "Excuse me, just another hot flash, it'll be gone in a moment." So, many women suffer in silence.

No one will refute the fact that estrogen usually combats hot flashes and myriad other symptoms of menopause, but the question remains: "Should I take estrogen?"

This book has been written to help you make that decision and to answer that question. It contains all the information currently available about estrogen, in both its pharmaceutical and plant forms. It makes no attempt to diagnose your situation, nor does it contain any prescriptions for you to follow. No book should do that. *The Estrogen Answer Book* is designed so that you can find easy-to-understand, comprehensive answers to your key question, and it is set up so that you can find answers to your other questions about estrogen easily and quickly. It is filled with pertinent information — which is sometimes reiterated, in case you don't read the book cover to cover on first reading.

Read on, learn what you need to know about estrogen, and determine whether or not it is for you. Share your thoughts about estrogen with your physician. Then you too can "get on with it."

Understanding the anatomy of menopause is an important first step in getting on with it. Long before we are born there are hormonal activities at work shaping us, preparing us for puberty, and even enabling us to reproduce. Women's primary female sex hormones are estrogen and progesterone. Even though we've also heard it called the male hormone, women also have a bit of testosterone, which is one of the androgen hormones.

At birth our ovaries contain all the eggs we will ever have, some 500,000, it is said. These eggs remain intact as we spend our early years nonreproductively. At puberty, however, which can occur as early as nine years of age or as late as thirteen or later, our estrogen production surges. Estrogen is produced by our ovaries, with a little coming also from our adrenal glands. With that surge at puberty, women enter the reproductive years of their lives, with the monthly cycling of estrogen, progesterone, and the resulting monthly menstrual period. This cycle typically continues unless interrupted by pregnancy (or by amenorrhea caused by illness, medication, or excessive exercise such as in the case of the elite athlete) until menopause, which occurs on average around the age of 51 years and 4 months. Then we enter our nonreproductive years.

It may well be that menopause is simply puberty in reverse. It is important to know what goes on in our bodies between our first and our last menstrual cycle. During all that time, some thirty-five years, depending on when we as individuals have our first period and when we have our last (which is actually what menopause represents), a complicated symphony has been playing chiefly between our brain and our ovaries. It begins when the hypothalamus gland, located at the base of the brain in the center of the skull, signals the pituitary gland, also located in the base of the skull, to produce two hormones, follicle-stimulating hormone (FSH) and luteinizing hormone (LH), that directly affect the growth and development of the ovarian follicle, the tiny sac that contains each egg. The FSH stimulates the follicle, causing it to ripen, and then the LH causes the egg to mature and be released from the follicle.

These two powerful glands, the hypothalamus and the pituitary, actually control our reproductive system. They stimulate the ovaries to secrete the female sex hormones estrogen and progesterone (and yes, that bit of testosterone as well), to prepare the lining of the uterus for a fertilized egg should a pregnancy occur. When there is no pregnancy that month, the lining is shed in what we know as our monthly menstrual period, and the cycle begins again.

Normally this cyclic rhythm continues throughout our reproductive years, perhaps interrupted by a pregnancy or one of the other reasons mentioned above. Sometime in our late thirties or early forties that rhythmic cycle begins to change. Our periods may become erratic, coming closer together or farther apart, or they may become heavier or lighter in flow. These quirky changes may indicate that we are entering the perimenopausal, the getting-ready-for-menopause, years, and we may find other changes as well. Those perimenopausal years used to be referred to as the "climacteric," from the Greek for "critical time."

Whatever its name, this time of change and changes is the result of our running out of our preprogrammed number of eggs. Eventually, no matter how hard the FSH and LH work they can no longer stimulate the ovary to produce an egg or the estrogen and progesterone hormones that follow, and we have arrived at menopause. The hard work of the FSH often shows up on the blood test you may have to determine whether you are entering menopause. For example, a blood test that shows that your FSH levels are higher than 40 mIU/ml (that means 40 milli international units per milliliter) tells you: "Hello, menopause has arrived." Now please note, this is the average way that women encounter menopause, but some women may run out of eggs much earlier than the average age and then encounter premature menopause, generally considered to be before the age of forty. Surgical menopause caused by the removal of the uterus and both ovaries (hysterectomy with a bilateral oophorectomy) may occur whenever that surgery is performed.

So here we stand, at menopause, on the brink of perhaps another thirty-five wonderful, productive — although nonreproductive — years. And so we must decide whether or not to replace those missing hormones — progesterone, a little testosterone perhaps, and estrogen — which is what this book is all about.

The Facts

PART ONE

1

What Is Estrogen?

SOME fifty million baby boomer women are now moving through the menopausal age range. They are entering at the rate of somewhere between 3,500 and 4,000 per day. Almost all still have questions about menopause and even more questions about estrogen. They want to know exactly what estrogen is and why it has such a profound effect on their bodies. Of course, most of them already know that it is one of the female sex hormones and that it affects most of their body's systems from birth to death. But why is estrogen so important that it needs to be replaced after menopause? To answer that question, let's review how our experience with estrogen begins.

Estrogen is a hormone that starts to work in your body in the years before puberty. That is when the brain begins sending messages via the hypothalamus, a small collection of specialized brain cells, to the pituitary gland nestled in its base and to the ovaries, telling them it is time to warm up for the exquisite symphony that will soon begin. The ovaries get ready. Eggs within them begin to mature, and with the advent of menstruation you know that an egg has matured enough to be released in the process called ovulation. The egg makes its way down one of the fallopian tubes to the uterus and, meeting no sperm coming the other way, is expelled in what became known as "the curse," your "period," "the monthlies," or whatever other nickname you used for menstruation.

The symphony plays beautifully for most women, its rhythm interrupted occasionally by a pregnancy, a profound passage in which estrogen is also assigned a significant role. Then women begin to experience some symphonic dissonance in their forties; some women even in their thirties or younger, although that is fairly uncommon. Even though they had not considered the value of the work in which their hormones were engaged in the past, some women become aware of changes. Some changes are subtle; others are profound. A hot flash or a night sweat creeps into their otherwise organized life, disturbing work, sleep, or a lover's tryst. Periods that were so regular that it was possible to plan vacations around them start coming closer together or farther apart and bleeding ranges from unusually little to way too much. It is a confusing and unsettling time. Often for women this change in estrogen and progesterone (the other major female sex hormone) production and the quirky symptoms that follow usher in the perimenopausal years, those years before your final period.

The important reference points here are the year before menstruation, when all systems were tuning up, and menopause, your final period. In the last decade, much has been written to explain menopause, its signs and its symptoms; not enough is known, however, about what to do when we pass through and want — perhaps need — to have the same hormonal protection of the perimenopausal years.

On average, menopause begins at age 51.4 months. Having said that, you can expect it anytime within a ten-year period between ages forty-five and fifty-five, which used to be referred to as the climacteric. The trouble with all these lines of demarcation is that they don't apply to all women. For example, eight out of a hundred women will go through menopause before age forty-five, some as early as their thirties or even their twenties. Although it is rare, I've interviewed women who are still waiting for menopause as they approach their sixtieth birthday.

We know that menopause is the culmination of a gradual process that begins three to five years before our last menstrual period. It occurs when our ovaries cease functioning and we have run out of eggs, and our estrogen and progesterone production system has diminished or shut down altogether. We know that menopause can also occur surgically — and suddenly — when we have a hysterectomy with a bilateral oophorectomy. We know that symptoms of menopause can range from the all-too-common hot flash and its twin, the night sweat, which can affect 75 to 85 percent of women, to rarer symptoms such as heel pains, dry mouth, and formication — from the Greek word *formica,* which means "ants." It describes perfectly that strange symptom that makes you feel like the creepy-crawlies are invading your skin.

What we don't know for sure and what we're having difficulty determining individually is "Should I take estrogen?" To help with your deliberations, it is important that you know everything there is to know about estrogen. So let's begin.

1   What is estrogen?

Everyone talks about what estrogen does, but few realize what estrogen really is. Estrogen is actually three different female sex hormones. Hormones are often called chemical messengers. They are chemicals produced by the endocrine glands or tissues, and they affect other organs. They influence growth, metabolism, sexual development, behavior, and other essential human processes. The three kinds of estrogen are *estradiol, estriol,* and *estrone.* The most powerful and constant of the three is estradiol, which is produced by the ovaries during each menstrual cycle. Estriol is produced in large amounts only during pregnancy, and estrone is the form of estrogen that is found in postmenopausal women, but in much smaller amounts than the amount of estradiol that circulates during a woman's reproductive years.

2   What part does estrogen play during the reproductive years?

Estrogen, in the form of estradiol, is produced following the release of an egg during the menstrual cycle. Its job is to thicken the lining of the uterus, called the endometrium, in case a pregnancy occurs. It also reports to the brain, telling it when to cut back on sending more follicle-stimulating hormone (FSH) and when to begin sending luteinizing hormone (LH). These hormones also play key roles in the cycle. Estrogen's main role is to control the functioning of the reproductive organs — the ovaries, uterus, breasts, and genitalia. But estrogen is also required by other organs of the body, such as the brain, blood vessels, bone, heart, liver, fat, muscles, and skin. Scientists have found estrogen receptors, little lock-sites that enable estrogens to get inside cells to exert their effects on all these organs and more. There are at least three hundred processes in the body that are affected by estrogen production that have little or nothing to do with the reproduction process. These will become apparent as we delve deeper into the many roles of estrogen.

3   What role does estrogen play in pregnancy?

A significant amount of estriol is secreted by the ovaries and the placenta during pregnancy. Some studies reveal that it may well be abnormally high levels of estriol that contribute to some of the complications of pregnancy, such as debilitating morning sickness. Other studies have shown that estriol may offer protection against breast cancer. Therapeutic estriol, made from the soybean plant, is difficult to find in the United States. It is available in Canada and Europe, and can be ordered by your physician through some compounding pharmacies. To research its availability, check with the National Association of Compounding Pharmacists, listed in appendix D. (Estrogen and breast cancer will be covered in chapter 4).

4   If estrogen, in the form of estrone, is the primary circulating hormone during the postmenopausal years, why is that not enough to protect my heart, bones, brain, and the rest of my body?

Estrone is a much weaker form of estrogen, and it is present at much lower levels than the estradiol circulating in your body during your reproductive years. It does not offer the same protection as estradiol, but it is the ingredient in some oral estrogen tablets. For example, Ogen, a replacement estrogen tablet produced by Pharmacia & Upjohn, contains estrone. Estrone is made in the fat cells of the body, so obese women, more than likely, have more estrone and fewer problems with hot flashes and other menopause symptoms. Estrone is actually made from androstenedione, a precursor hormone of testosterone manufactured by the adrenal glands, those small glands located on top of each kidney. The adrenal glands secrete the androgen hormones and small amounts of estrogen and progesterone. The androgens are the hormones that produce male characteristics and are largely responsible for libido in women and men. Yes, women have testosterone, too, but in much smaller amounts than men.

5 What are hormones, in general?

Hormones are chemical messengers secreted by various glands in the body. They are specifically programmed to perform certain acts. For example, once a hormone is released into the bloodstream, it may go directly to a "target" gland, telling the target gland to produce its own hormone; or the original hormone, once circulating, may have been programmed to set off chemical reactions in different parts of the body. Your body makes literally dozens of different hormones, which regulate functions related to most systems of the body. For example, some hormones assist the body in managing stress by regulating blood flow to certain organs and by regulating the tension of our muscles. These hormones are important to our "fight or flight" instincts when we are faced with stressful situations.

6 What is progesterone?

Progesterone is also a female sex hormone, and is produced by the corpus luteum of the ovary. Its role is to bring tissues to maturity and limit their growth. For example, we know that one of the tasks assigned to estrogen is to thicken the lining of the uterus should a pregnancy occur. Progesterone, on the other hand, has as one of its routine jobs to prevent the lining of the uterus (called the endometrium) from growing to the point where it causes excessively heavy or long-lasting menstrual bleeding. In

the case of a pregnancy, progesterone triggers nutrient-laden se-
cretions important to the fertilized egg as it moves through the
fallopian tube and adheres to the uterine lining. Progesterone also
has a profound effect upon certain cells, such as helping the
breasts get their milk production system ready for nursing the
new baby. When the ovaries run out of eggs, causing menopause,
the production of progesterone, like that of estrogen, diminishes
and often ceases altogether.

7   How do estrogen and progesterone work?

Estrogen and progesterone both have significant effects
on many of the body's chemical and physical functions, but they
may either work together or work in opposition. A good example
of the opposing effect of these hormones can be seen in the nervous system, where estrogen may be viewed as an "upper" because of its mental tonic effect while progesterone can be a
"downer," causing feelings of deep fatigue and minor depression,
or the blues. These opposing effects result for a number of reasons. Estrogen stimulates the nervous system; progesterone acts
as a sedative on it. Estrogen tends to lower blood sugar levels;
progesterone elevates them. An appropriate, healthy balance between these two female hormones is vitally important. We'll discover even more about them in later chapters, when we discuss
replacing hormones after menopause.

8   Once released, how does estrogen make its way into other cells of the body?

"Estrogen receptors" permit estrogen to enter cells. The
best way to visualize a receptor is as a lock on a cell. Think of
estrogen holding the key. As estrogen circulates through the body
it is able to turn the key on these locks, or estrogen receptors,
and enter the cell as a messenger, causing the cell to perform
whatever function or functions it has been programmed to do.
Exciting new research findings have revealed that there are two
kinds of receptors on cells: alpha receptors, which permit estrogen

to enter the cell and perform its function there, and beta receptors, which keep estrogen locked out. From this recent research will come new and perhaps improved methods of administering estrogen replacement therapy.

9   What are "designer estrogens"?

Currently we are faced with the exciting prospect of being able to use estrogen selectively, because it can be designed to enter some cells and be locked out of others. That is how the term "designer estrogens" began to be bandied about in the media. The new class of pharmaceutical estrogens is technically called Selective Estrogen Receptor Modulators, or SERMs for short. For example, one SERM that was recently approved by the Food and Drug Administration (FDA) is a synthetic estrogen compound called raloxifene. It is a product of Eli Lilly and Company and is available by prescription under the name of Evista. Studies have shown that raloxifene can enter bone cells, helping to prevent osteoporosis, while it remains locked out of breast and uterus cells. Another product, called droloxifene, under study by Pfizer Laboratories, may do the same. There are another six similar products, and maybe even more, being researched by other laboratories right now. It is believed that these new products, these SERMs of one kind or another, will protect against breast and uterine cancer while preventing osteoporosis and heart disease and perhaps other illnesses as well.

Evista does prevent osteoporosis, and it has positive effects on blood lipids, but it is not quite as effective in these respects as the estrogen products already in use, such as Premarin. But Evista signals the beginning of a new kind of estrogen replacement therapy for women who have had or who fear breast cancer. Evista does not limit or diminish other menopausal symptoms, such as the common hot flash and its twin, the night sweat, nor does it repair vaginal dryness. More about Evista appears throughout this book and more specifically in chapter 8

It is clearly too early to know what place SERMs will take

in the armamentarium of women's postmenopausal options, but surely they will add an important new dimension. However, we all know too well that wonder drugs must stand the test of time.

10   How does estrogen affect the body?

Estrogen enters the cells of different tissues of the body and causes physiological changes by stimulating chemical reactions. As explained earlier, estrogen has an effect on literally hundreds of processes in the body. Some of its most important effects include the following: Estrogen has an important effect on the heart, protecting women from developing heart attacks and strokes by elevating the high-density lipoprotein or HDL (the "good" cholesterol) and lowering the low-density lipoprotein or LDL (the "bad" cholesterol) and by keeping the lining of the blood vessels pliant and flexible. Estrogen prevents osteoporosis by helping us to maintain bone mineral density, necessary for strong, healthy bones. Estrogen plumps up and fills out our skin; and it has distinct and positive effects on our heart, bladder, and myriad other organs as well as on our brain, affecting our mind, our mood, and our memory.

2

Should I Take Estrogen?

HOULD I take estrogen replacement therapy (ERT)?
Should I be on hormone replacement therapy (HRT)?
Those are the really big questions for most women experiencing the early stages of the menopause transition, and the
deliberations can go on endlessly. Women actually find themselves dividing into camps whenever the subject arises. There are
those who wouldn't be without their replacement hormones,
those who won't even consider taking them, and — the largest
group — those for whom the situation remains confusing and
who are uncertain about what to do. Unfortunately, too many
women remain essentially uninformed about the range of choices
they have when it comes to replacing estrogen, and the fact that
whatever decision they make need not be forever.

But, before we go any further, let me define ERT and HRT.
Throughout this book references are made to estrogen replacement therapy (ERT) and hormone replacement therapy (HRT).
ERT refers to the use of estrogen alone. HRT refers to the use of
estrogen and progestin or estrogen and progesterone, which is
usually prescribed for women with an intact uterus to safeguard
them against endometrial cancer.

That women have all these choices and decisions is a relatively new turn of events. At the turn of the last century, women's
lives ended just about or even a little earlier than their time of
menopause, which, you recall, averages about age fifty-one.

Women who lived beyond the menopause were considered to be old and often considered themselves old and, therefore, deserving of the "miseries" of age.

There were some very early attempts to give women injections of various sorts of estrogenic animal preparations to quell menopause symptoms, but these were not widely used or scientifically recognized. Then, in 1939, Ayerst, McKenna and Harrison, a Canadian pharmaceutical company, in cooperation with J. B. Collip, Ph.D., a pioneer in endocrinology research at McGill University in Montreal, made a breakthrough in the process of extracting estrogen from pregnant mares' urine. In 1942 Premarin, as it came to be named, was approved for use in the United States.

In 1966 a book called *Feminine Forever*, written by a Brooklyn, New York, gynecologist, Robert A. Wilson, promised women eternal youth through estrogen. This book had a profound influence on the extent to which estrogen was prescribed in the United States, Europe, and elsewhere. Though some accuse Dr. Wilson of being a savvy salesman for the pharmaceutical companies, I rather doubt that he holds that dubious distinction. Rather, I see him as a pioneer, opening up the subject of menopause and the changes women undergo at midlife and offering women the knowledge that help with estrogen was available and that they might get that help from their physicians. If this did, indeed, also open the doors to the medicalization of menopause, it also created a stir in the research community, which for far too long had turned a deaf ear to women's problems.

Sales of estrogen to treat menopause symptoms such as hot flashes, mood swings, and vaginal dryness increased swiftly, until suddenly two articles in the *New England Journal of Medicine* in December 1976 brought them almost to a halt. The articles reported a strong association between estrogen replacement therapy and endometrial cancer (cancer of the lining of the uterus). Women were pulled off estrogen abruptly, my own mother among them. I remember her angst at that development and her search for something else to make her feel as good as she had on estrogen. Nothing did. The fountain of youth was stilled. But not for long.

In the early 1980s physicians began to prescribe estrogen with progestin (synthetic progesterone), which would mimic the way your own body would produce and cycle those two hormones if your ovarian production system were still functioning. The thinking was then, and is today, that a woman with an intact uterus could benefit from the estrogen while being protected from endometrial cancer by the progestin. Although some scientific thinking still concludes that estrogen with progestin provides a safer approach, many women and some physicians remain cautious about the use of estrogen. For example, today perhaps 20 percent of postmenopausal women in the United States use estrogen, although that number appears to be slowly growing.

It is interesting to note that over the years I have come across women who somehow managed to stay on estrogen even during the '70s scare. One woman, now well into her eighties, whose looks belie her years, reports none of the problems women associate with aging and insists that if her own physician had not gone along with her urgent request to stay on estrogen, she would have found one who would have agreed to her demand.

Women today want and need to make smart choices for themselves too. They are educated, interested, and accustomed to asking questions and getting answers. They read books and magazine articles, and show up at health education seminars in ever increasing numbers. Women want to know about midlife perimenopausal and menopausal changes, and how those might affect them both physiologically and psychologically. They want to know what to do about the changes, in order to help themselves live not only longer but better lives.

Numerous studies throughout the world are trying to answer the myriad questions, the most important of which is the Women's Health Initiative (WHI), established by the National Institutes of Health Office on Women's Health Research. It is hoped when completed in 2005 the WHI will give women many of the answers. That project is both exciting and daunting. Most women want answers today. The year 2005 will be too late for some of us. Further, the conclusions of most studies seem to be written on shifting sand. Every study seems to send other researchers back to their laboratories to refute, change, or add to what has been found or is known. That scientific method may inch research forward, but it doesn't do much for a woman today who wants the answer to her question, "Should I take estrogen?"

11 **I'm thirty-eight years old. I just learned that I have to undergo a hysterectomy with a bilateral oophorectomy (removal of both ovaries). My physician says I'll begin surgical menopause almost immediately, and he wants to put me on estrogen right after the procedure. Why should I take estrogen?**

Surgical menopause is the result of removal of your uterus and both ovaries and you are much too young for menopause. Let me explain. As you know, the average age for menopause is fifty-one. That's when women's ovaries run out of eggs and cease their production of the female hormones, estrogen and progesterone. Estrogen bathes and nourishes many of our organs and tissues and aids their processes. Since you will be losing your main source of estrogen too early, it is important for you to replace it so as not to be deprived of its protective effects many years earlier than you would have been naturally. Estrogen is vitally important for younger women; some studies show that along with other menopausal symptoms that may occur, some young women may develop depression within three years after this surgical procedure is performed. Although the depression is psychological, its roots are often physiological in origin. In addition, rather than the gradual process by which menopause usually arrives, the onset of surgical menopause is usually sudden, with full-blown symptoms. Taking estrogen will offset the onset of symptoms. (More about hysterectomy appears in chapter 13.)

12 My mother is seventy-two and bent over from osteoporosis. I am fifty-two and my physician says I should start taking estrogen now. How will estrogen help me avoid my mother's fate?

Prevention of osteoporosis has been described in many ways over the past decade, but none better, I think, than this: Think of osteoporosis prevention as a three-legged stool. One leg represents exercise — weight-bearing, of course; the second leg represents calcium, 1,000 to 1,500 milligrams a day, depending on your age; and the third leg represents estrogen replacement. It takes all three legs to make a sturdy stool. It takes all three legs to help you avoid your family history of osteoporosis, as well. (More information about osteoporosis appears in chapter 3.)

13 Hot flashes are dragging me down. Should I consider taking estrogen?

Hot flashes are vasomotor symptoms caused by changes in the chemistry of the brain, which begins a series of activities that can be likened to a domino effect. The chemical changes in the brain are the direct result of an abrupt drop in the body's production of estrogen. These chemical changes in the brain affect the temperature control center in the hypothalamus gland, which is also located in the brain. As a result, the hypothalamus directs the release of hormones that cause a decrease in the body's core temperature set point. That decrease, in turn, causes the blood vessels of the skin to dilate, and sweating results as your body — accustomed to its own set point — begins working to reset its thermostat. This entire disturbance makes you feel as if your internal thermostat has gone awry. Since it is the abrupt drop in the body's production of estrogen that starts the whole series of events, replacing that estrogen will usually stop hot flashes altogether.

Hot flashes can range widely, from simply being an annoyance to being desperately debilitating. A flash usually begins just above the waist and spreads upward, enveloping the chest, back, neck, face, and scalp. Some women have very few hot flashes, just a couple a day for a couple of years, while other women report having as many as fifty hot flashes a day for many years. Although it has not been scientifically proven, many women report relief from hot flashes with the use of vitamin E, in amounts that range between 400 international units (IU) and 1,000 IU per day. Check vitamin E with your physician before taking large amounts. Limiting stress, alcohol, caffeine, and spicy foods is also a good idea; they can set off hot flashes in some women. Other women report having cold flashes, which seem to subside with the use of estrogen as well. Dressing in layers is a good option in either event.

14 **I've been taking birth control pills for years. Once I cross over into menopause should I start taking estrogen, and what's the difference between the estrogen in "the pill" and the estrogen used in replacement therapy?**

Even the new low-dose birth control pills contain a significantly greater amount of estrogen than the doses typically prescribed to counteract postmenopausal symptoms. It seems you have no problem tolerating birth control pills, and you may be one of the lucky women who simply slide into menopause, change your estrogen source and amount, and experience nary a symptom. I say lucky, because it wasn't too many years ago that physicians made women wait until they had gone one full year without a period before they would prescribe ERT or HRT, no matter how badly their symptoms affected them. The new low-dose minipills changed that philosophy, but the switch can be tricky. Part of the reason doctors wanted women to wait that full year was to be sure that their estrogen was depleted and their reproductive lives had definitely come to a close, before adding replacement estrogen to the amount they might normally have had. This was risky business, because just thinking you couldn't become pregnant didn't always work. Many a surprise bundle of joy was conceived during that interim. In addition, if you were still producing estrogen, adding more might have caused other problems.

When the time comes, check with your physician to learn whether you are through the menopause and ready to change the source and lessen the amount of your estrogen product and change your regimen. A simple blood test, or several blood tests, if one is not conclusive, will usually give you the answer.

15 Does every woman need estrogen?

Various expert sources offer differing answers to that question — and that's not very helpful, I know. Some physicians say that up to one-third of women do not need estrogen, indicating that perhaps they have some compensatory mechanism enabling their own bodies to produce the amount of estrogen they require. Some postmenopausal women seem able to produce a small but sufficient amount of estrogen or to convert other hormones in the body to estrogen. Other women are able to use the estrogen stored in their fatty tissues, compensating to some degree for the ovaries' stoppage of estrogen production. Often these are the women who seem to sail right through menopause with neither a symptom nor a complaint. I say *seem* to sail through, because unless they know the condition of their bones and how the rest of their organs that require estrogen's protection are faring, how do they know if they are sailing through or whether they are simply symptom free for the present?

Women who have risk factors for certain illnesses such as osteoporosis and heart disease (we'll discuss those factors in chapter 4) and women whose symptoms are uncomfortable, as well as those women who have no medical reason not to take estrogen, often choose to do so. For example, the four out of ten postmenopausal women who will ultimately have osteoporosis probably need to learn as early in their lives as possible that they are at high risk. The three-legged stool mentioned earlier might be what they need to stand straight and tall upon. But some women simply cannot take estrogen, for medical reasons, and those will be described in chapter 4.

16   Will estrogen make me gain weight?

This is a fairly common concern, and the answer from a recent study says no. Yet a side effect of HRT or ERT often seems to be a small amount of weight gain. Or weight gain may be a factor of menopause and of just getting older. We live in a society that is frantic to remain or become thin. Concerning estrogen and weight gain, I have uncovered various reports, some indicating that water retention and bloating can account for perhaps four to six pounds showing on the scale when taking estrogen — no more than that. This new study, reported in the *Journal of Clinical Endocrinology and Metabolism*, May 1997, showed that postmenopausal women using hormone replacement therapy actually had slightly less average weight gain than women who took placebos. The study provides evidence that women should not be deterred from starting HRT or ERT for fear of weight gain. If anything, the study demonstrated that replacement therapy might slightly blunt a tendency for some postmenopausal women to put on excess pounds.

Other studies demonstrate clearly that the changes in our metabolism that begin around the age of thirty-five are at fault for weight gain. It is then that our metabolism begins to slow down between 1/2 and 1 percent per year. It's when we should begin revving up our exercise programs and slowing down our calorie consumption. Let me explain why we need to do this. Say, for example, that your metabolism is slowing down at the rate of 1 percent per year. In the fifteen or so years between age thirty-five and when you reach the average age for menopause, your metabolism will have slowed down some 15 percent. To offset that slowdown you must make some minor changes in your lifestyle. You must eat more healthful foods and reduce portions, and exercise more. I know some women who practically pray to the bathroom scale each morning for a favorable reading. If they get the right answer, they have a good day. Otherwise, they feel defeated.

A woman caught up with me after my lecture a few months

ago and said, "The problem with this whole menopause and estrogen business that you've been talking about is that it's got me divided in half. I think of myself as Victoria I, the former me with the flat stomach, and Victoria II, the postmenopausal, estrogen-taking me with the high, rounded stomach. I want Victoria I back, but I just can't seem to find her." From my vantage point, Victoria is a shapely, well-dressed woman in her mid to late fifties who looks terrific, healthy and well toned. So I said to her, "You look great, you tell me you feel great, so why not wake up each morning and just tell your tummy that you love it. It's a better way to start your day."

17   Should I take progesterone with estrogen, and if so, why?

Current scientific thinking is that if your uterus is intact you should take both hormones. The "why" goes back to the situation described earlier, following the publication of Dr. Wilson's book, *Feminine Forever*, which took the country by storm and inaugurated the estrogen replacement revolution. At that time estrogen alone was prescribed. Then those two articles in 1976 in the prestigious *New England Journal of Medicine*, reporting cancer of the uterus in women taking estrogen, abruptly stopped the revolution. The articles clearly demonstrated a strong association between estrogen replacement therapy and the development of endometrial (uterine) cancer. For several years most women patients were not offered estrogen by their rightfully conservative physicians. What happened then in the early '80s was that physicians began to prescribe estrogen with progestin, which mimics the way your own body produces those two female hormones when your ovaries are still functioning. Many physicians believed then, and most continue to believe today, that a woman whose uterus is intact can obtain all the benefits of estrogen if she also takes progestin to protect her from endometrial cancer. You will recall that it is the progestin that causes the lining of the uterus to shed in what we know as our menstrual flow (see question 58 in chapter 4 for discussion of "menstruating forever"). With no buildup of the lining of the uterus, the endometrium does not become thickened or precancerous. Today there are many regimens for using both hormones, and those are described in chapter 7.

18 **Do I really need to replace the estrogen that I lose after menopause?**

Good question, difficult answer. The answer for each woman has to be individually tailored. Full knowledge and awareness of your medical history and your family members' medical histories are pertinent. For example, do you have hereditary risk factors for osteoporosis or heart disease or for some of the other diseases that studies have demonstrated can benefit from estrogen's protective effect, such as colon/rectal cancer, Alzheimer's disease, or osteoarthritis? Do you yourself have few or perhaps even no risk factors for these illnesses? If not, perhaps you do not need to consider replacing estrogen for now. I say "for now" because each new study, as I see it, seems to add to the growing list of benefits for women who can and want to take estrogen. No matter what you do now, I suggest you keep an open mind and periodically revisit this subject. But before you decide, this question really needs to be repeated in your own physician's office. Go in armed with as much information as you can. Take the Estrogen Decision Self-Evaluation "Test" at the end of chapter 14 to help you prepare.

19 **What tests will be ordered by my physician to determine whether estrogen is for me?**

Before prescribing estrogen, your physician will take, or review, if it's been done earlier, your family medical history and your personal history, looking primarily for information about cancer, heart disease, and osteoporosis. Undoubtedly, you will then have a full physical including a breast exam and a pelvic with a Pap test. A mammogram will probably be ordered at this time and, I would hope, a bone density test and an electrocardiogram as well. Your blood pressure will be checked. Usually, blood is drawn for a full battery of tests that include checking out serum estradiol levels, liver function, cholesterol and triglyceride levels, thyroid function, blood sugar (glucose) levels, and phosphorus and calcium levels. When the results of all these tests are back, your physician should review them with you and tell you whether he or she feels you should take estrogen or not. This is a good time for you to learn your physician's position on ERT, and what has determined that position. That information will enable you then to make your best decision concerning estrogen. Remember, it is unfair to yourself to decide what to do without having the benefit of all this information.

Even with all that information, some physicians, before starting you on estrogen, or on estrogen and progesterone if you have an intact uterus, will also perform a vaginal ultrasound or an endometrial biopsy to check out the condition of the lining of your uterus, making sure there are no abnormal cells harboring there. Another test sometimes performed is the "progesterone challenge test," whereby you take 10 milligrams of progesterone for seven to ten days. When you are done, you should bleed if there is adequate estrogen in your system. If you don't bleed, it may mean your estrogen levels are low, and starting HRT would be appropriate.

20 Should I start estrogen now or hang on without it for as long as I can?

Here again all the symptoms and all the risk factors come into play. Are your periods quirky — closer together, farther apart, heavier or lighter? Or have you stopped menstruating altogether? If your answer to either question is yes, you might want to see your physician for a follicle-stimulating hormone test. That simple blood test will be used to determine the ratio of FSH to estradiol in your system. If the FSH number is higher than 40 and your estradiol is lower than 14, estrogen replacement therapy may well be in the offing for you. This is true also if you are suffering debilitating symptoms such as hot flashes, night sweats, insomnia, palpitations, minor depression, mood swings, anxiety, joint pain, fatigue, vaginal dryness, or other symptoms that have undermined the quality of your life. High risk for the diseases that estrogen may prevent would also be a good reason for beginning estrogen therapy. When I lecture or write, I always suggest that each woman read everything she can about menopause and about estrogen, so she can make the best decision for herself.

21 Can I stop taking estrogen at any time?

You can, but I strongly suggest you discuss your decision with your physician first. As you know, estrogen and progesterone are powerful hormones, so should you decide to discontinue either HRT or ERT, it is important that you do so gradually. Discuss your reasons for discontinuing therapy: if your medication is not ridding you of uncomfortable symptoms, or your blood pressure is up, or you feel bloated and are concerned because you've gained a few pounds. Most women do not realize that there are many different estrogen preparations, many different dosages, and several different regimens for taking estrogen (all of which I will discuss in later chapters). Perhaps another product, dose, or way of taking it would solve your problems and you could continue to benefit from estrogen.

However, if ERT is not for you, taper off the medication slowly. Physicians often suggest the following schedule for weaning off the oral tablet: Take tablets for day 1 and day 2. Skip day 3. Take tablets on days 4 and 5. Skip day 6. And so forth for about two weeks. Then the next week take one tablet every other day, and finally, 1/2 tablet every other day for a week or so and then stop.

The patch (see chapter 5) is a little more complicated. Physicians have suggested either putting clear tape across half of the surface of the patch that goes next to your body, so that you will be absorbing only half of your dose, or cutting the patch in half and taping its edges to achieve the same decrease in dosage. Continue changing your altered patches in the same routine as you had before for the first two weeks; change once a week for the second two weeks, and then stop altogether.

In these ways, your body has a chance of getting used to going without estrogen. In her book *Women's Bodies, Women's Wisdom,* Dr. Christiane Northrup suggests that if you wish to come off estrogen you do it very slowly over a six-month period, to allow your body time to readjust. Her system seems the simplest. Each month you drop one pill. For example, the first month you stop taking a pill on Mondays. The second month on Mondays and Tuesdays, and so forth until you're done. But before you make *any* changes, do discuss stopping estrogen with your own physician, who not only needs to know what you are doing but who might also have a better system for discontinuing therapy.

22 What should I do if my physician doesn't believe in prescribing ERT or HRT?

Ask your doctor the reasons behind his or her attitudes toward ERT and HRT, and discuss them in detail. Ask whether that is her or his general belief, and pertains to all patients in the practice, or if this decision applies specifically to you. If the decision is because of your risk factors or your medical condition, ask for a complete explanation and make sure you are comfortable with the doctor's reasoning. If it is the physician's general policy to avoid estrogen and you want to try it, ask for a referral to a practitioner who might be able to help you. You can also check with a hospital or the medical society in your area for referral. Most often, they will provide you with the names of two or three physicians who can fit the bill. Also check with family members and friends, and from all these sources determine which name or names of physicians are mentioned repeatedly. Make consulting appointments with the top two physicians on your list, one or both of whom should be able to help you make your decision. Another good option is to write to the North American Menopause Society (see appendix D) and ask for the names of physicians in your area who have registered with them and indicated that they treat women going through menopause.

When it comes to taking estrogen, there is much information to gather and many decisions to be made . . . none irrevocable.

3

What Are the Benefits of Estrogen Replacement Therapy?

E VEN with the vast number of books, articles, lectures, and seminars about menopause during the last decade, according to more than 70 percent of the women who fill out my questionnaires, most women still want to know more about menopause — and a lot more about estrogen. Will ERT benefit me? They continue to ask.

The nature of their questions hasn't changed much over the past few years, with more than 64 percent of women surveyed wanting more knowledge about the psychological effects of menopause and over 62 percent desiring additional information about the physiological effects. Concerns about weight gain are up there near the top of the list, just under 60 percent, and anxiety, irritability, and mood swings run just about neck-and-neck at slightly over 58 percent. Other questions persist when it comes to insomnia (50.5 percent), minor depression (46.4 percent), vaginal dryness (44.9 percent), hot flashes (40.2 percent), and waning sexual libido (38.9 percent).

When I review the questions that are brought forward at programs and workshops, I see that they, too, haven't changed much over the past few years. There is undoubtedly at least a twofold reason for this: First, the audiences keep changing as more and more women enter the menopausal age range. Second, as postmenopausal women realize that they are living longer they themselves want to check out estrogen, even though they might never have been offered it or because they had not chosen to take it at an earlier time.

Now the number of estrogen choices is confounding. To start with, you can choose the kind of estrogen you may wish to try. There are tablets such as Premarin, produced by Wyeth-Ayerst, that represent the gold standard, having been around and tested for more than fifty-five years. Then there are patches. Patch therapy first became available with FDA approval of a transdermal system called Estraderm, made by Ciba Geigy (now Novartis Pharmaceutical). Today there are all kinds of patches on the market, such as Vivelle, also made by Novartis; Climara, produced by Berlex Laboratories; and the newest, Fempatch, by Parke-Davis. Just last year, Pharmacia & Upjohn Pharmaceuticals introduced Estring, an estrogen system through which a ring of estrogen is placed directly into the vagina in a manner similar to the diaphragm used as a contraceptive device. Estring, which is designed for postmenopausal urogenital symptoms, is available now with a prescription from your physician. A review of these and other products appears in chapter 5.

Today there is a vast array of doses that may work for you, since most products come in several different strengths. There are also different regimens to try if you have an intact uterus and need to take both estrogen and progestin. Both cycling and continuous regimens will be discussed in chapter 7.

If you wish to take estrogen, there is a long list of benefits that you might reap. There are risks as well, and these will be covered in chapter 4. But starting with the benefits seems most logical, since if you have chosen to read this book you are already considering estrogen and wondering whether it will be of benefit to you.

I have watched the tide turn concerning estrogen since the publication of *Managing Your Menopause* in 1990, a book I co-authored. I have paid attention to each study as it came along and tried to attend many of the scientific meetings at which the subject of estrogen was central. All of this activity only served to solidify my position that estrogen is important for women *if* there is no medical condition that precludes taking it. R. Jeffrey Chang, M.D., director of reproductive endocrinology and infertility at University of California, San Diego, School of Medicine, has said, "I think that in general across the board all women who lack estrogen should consider taking estrogen. The problem, I believe, is that women simply don't know enough about the reasons that they should take estrogen."

In this chapter we're going to look at those reasons, to help you decide whether estrogen can help you. Yes, I know, many women have the sense that they don't wish to put something foreign into their bodies. I must remind you that estrogen is not foreign to us: it began circulating in our bloodstream, providing its benefits to more than three hundred body processes, in the years just before puberty. Other women indicate that they don't wish to mess with Mother Nature. Perhaps we ought to look at it a different way, since Mother Nature has messed with us. I remind women time and again that the last time a century turned, our lives ended at just about the same time as our reproductive lives. Women did not need to make an estrogen decision then.

Today a healthy woman at fifty-one, the average age for menopause, is only halfway through her adult life. So with another half ahead, she may well want to consider replacing estrogen. But medical and scientific inconsistencies on the subject of estrogen, and the subsequent blasts in the news media each time a pro or con study is reported, make it very difficult for women to know what to do. Is the answer to estrogen replacement a conundrum? As one woman questioned during one of my recent seminars, "Ruth, are you telling me to take estrogen to protect myself from osteoporosis in my eighties and heart disease in my seventies, so that I can get breast cancer in my fifties?" No, I'm not!

However, therein lies the crux of the dilemma. Although I must admit that studies concerning estrogen and breast cancer continue to confuse and confound us, I believe that with the complete information known to date about the benefits and the risks of taking estrogen, each woman will have an easier time making her own estrogen decision. I think this book is important, because each time as I look around an auditorium when I am speaking, more than ever before I see women who represent an ever widening range of ages. That indicates to me that for many women the jury is still out when it comes to finalizing their personal estrogen decision. Since I am always asked this question first, I think we should begin with understanding where some of our physicians stand on the important issue of estrogen replacement therapy.

23 What is the main reason that physicians prescribe estrogen?

I sincerely believe that physicians, cognizant of our longer life spans and our escalating risk factors as we age, choose to prescribe estrogen so that women can live better while they are living longer. Although HRT and ERT are much maligned as tools of the pharmaceutical industry's march to medicalize menopause and market them, I don't believe for one minute that physicians suggest estrogen for any reason other than the best interests of the patient. Having said that, I must add that too many physicians do not have, or take, the time to tell their patients why they want to prescribe estrogen for them and to discuss the choices women have in product, dosage, and regimen. Sadly, this lack of information and give-and-take discussion leads to unfilled prescriptions or the decisions women make to stop therapy without discussing it with their doctors.

24 Is estrogen a good choice for preventing osteoporosis?

You bet it is — along with a calcium-rich diet and weight-bearing exercise.

Menopause is a marker for rapid bone loss, and all postmenopausal women are at risk for osteoporosis (weakened bones). One out of two women past the age of menopause will eventually sustain an osteoporotic fracture. In fact, osteoporosis is the fourth leading killer of women and has rightfully been tagged as a woman's disease. According to National Osteoporosis

Foundation (NOF) statistics, 28 million Americans have osteo-porosis or are at risk of developing it: 10 million already have the disease, and 18 million have low bone mass, placing them at risk. Of these numbers, 80 percent are women.

Other pertinent new statistics from NOF include the fol-lowing:

- 90 percent of hip fractures and 90 percent of spine fractures in elderly white women are caused by osteoporosis;
- 80 percent of hip fractures and 80 percent of spine fractures in elderly black women are caused by osteoporosis;
- in other racial groups, well over half of hip and spine fractures are caused by osteoporosis;
- health care costs for treating osteoporotic fractures amount to $13.8 billion annually.

Even though osteoporosis is highlighted in the news these days, it is an old illness. Osteoporosis has been medically under-stood since the early 1940s and its risk factors have been known for a very long time.

Every time I see women with dowager's hump (dorsal ky-phosis), I am reminded of the toll osteoporosis takes on women's lives. Do you need to worry about this?

Yes you do, particularly if you have risk factors for the dis-ease. Review the risk factors listed in the answer to the next ques-tion and then consider: Your lifetime risk of breaking a hip due to osteoporosis is greater than your combined risk of developing breast, uterine, and ovarian cancer. Osteoporosis is a preventable disease, yet it still stands fourth on the National Institutes of Health's list of the leading causes of death in women, following heart disease, cancer, and stroke. To attack your fear of osteo-porosis, first have a bone density test, then, depending on the test's results and your risk factors, discuss with your physician a plan for preventing osteoporosis. Certainly, that discussion should include weight-bearing exercise, a calcium-rich diet, and estrogen.

25   What are the risk factors for osteoporosis?

The risk factors for osteoporosis are many and varied. As with other diseases, you can consider yourself lucky if you've "picked" the right parents. So, naturally, heredity heads the list of risk factors:

- family history of the disease
- early menopause (before age forty-five)
- being Caucasian or Asian
- having a sedentary lifestyle (that means you don't get much exercise)
- being fair, small boned, and thin
- having a lifelong low calcium intake
- long-term use or high doses of certain medications, including corticosteroids, heparin, anticonvulsants, and some chemotherapy drugs
- use of thyroid medication in excess of your needs (have an annual blood test to check it out)
- excessive use of alcohol, caffeine, protein, and colas (although some of these are debated from time to time)
- smoking

26   How can I check my bone health?

Many different kinds of tests are available for checking the strength of your bones. I sincerely believe that every woman at menopause or with a number of risk factors for osteoporosis should have a bone density test. Your test results may weigh heavily in your decision whether or not to take estrogen. Sadly, many women are still unaware that they should have such a test, and many physicians have not as yet incorporated bone density tests into their routine menopause examination procedures. Today some insurance companies are more willing to pay for bone density testing, and just last year a bill was passed making coverage by Medicare mandatory beginning July 1998. I keep thinking that general osteoporosis screening might be a good idea, but it hasn't been a popular one. Even though bone mineral density screening for osteoporosis is controversial because of its high cost, a Swedish study reported in the *Archives of Internal Medicine* in October 1997 indicated that screening had increased HRT and ERT use, especially in women with very low bone-mineral density.

A procedure called dual energy X-ray absorptiometry (DEXA) is the gold standard of bone density testing. It provides hip and spine bone measurements, takes fewer than fifteen minutes (the newest machine takes only eight minutes) to perform, and delivers less radiation than a standard chest X-ray or a dental X-ray. There's a fairly new portable ultrasound unit, called Achilles, from Lunar that measures the bone density in the heel; you place your heel for one minute in the heated water in the unit to get a reading. And the newest of all is a testing device approved by the FDA in March 1998, called Sahara by Hologic, Inc., which also measures bone density in the heel quickly but without the water, as the name implies. Other new testing procedures also look interesting. Discuss options with your physician. Whichever test you take, make *sure* you get tested.

27   What can I take if I do show bone loss?

Some estrogen products, like Premarin, are approved by the FDA for both prevention and treatment of osteoporosis; others just for prevention. Until recently, estrogen was the main medication for women with osteoporosis. Today there are also nonhormonal products, such as alendronate (Fosamax, a tablet), a product of Merck Laboratories, and calcitonin (Miacalcin, a form of salmon calcitonin available by injection and more recently as a nasal spray, manufactured by Sandoz Pharmaceutical) that slow bone breakdown. There are, as usual, side effects that you need to be aware of, such as digestive upset and esophageal irritation with Fosamax, which can be avoided if it is taken exactly as directed. It is suggested that you take Fosamax in the morning at least thirty minutes before eating or drinking anything other than eight ounces of plain water and then that you remain upright (standing or sitting) until the half hour has passed.

A recent study involving 1,609 healthy women ages forty-five to fifty-nine and at least six months postmenopausal was conducted at four medical centers to determine the effect of alendronate on postmenopausal women. It found that alendronate prevents bone loss in postmenopausal women under sixty years of age to nearly the same extent as estrogen-progestin. The study was reported in *The New England Journal of Medicine* February 19, 1998. So, another alternative for maintaining bone mass and reducing the risk of fractures in the future is available to women who do not need to control other symptoms of menopause with estrogen or who cannot or will not, for whatever reason, consider HRT or ERT.

Miacalcin, a salmon-calcitonin nasal spray, is often recommended for women five or more years past menopause who cannot or choose not to take estrogen. Miacalcin can cause mild nasal irritation, which is usually temporary.

Another product that quickly wended its way through the FDA approval process is the synthetic estrogen compound called raloxifene. Now approved and named Evista, this is the first of what I believe will be a whole string of "designer estrogens" that will become available for osteoporosis prevention and/or osteoporosis treatment indications. Evista is described in detail in chapter 8.

Sodium fluoride, not yet approved by the FDA for general use, is unlike the other products in that it actually stimulates bone formation. In the current study it is administered by slow-release tablet twice each day for one full year. Treatment then is discontinued for two months and then resumed. Sodium fluoride actually stimulates osteoblasts, the little Pac-Man–like critters that trigger bone formation.

All these preventives and treatments are bone saving, but should be used *along with* a calcium-rich diet — at least 1,000 milligrams of calcium daily, plus 400 IUs of vitamin D — and a regular routine of weight-bearing exercise.

28 Does ERT decrease my risk for developing cardiovascular problems?

That certainly is clear from many current studies, the most well known of which is the Harvard Nurses' Health Study, which has led investigators to conclude that women who take estrogen appear to have about half the risk of both fatal and nonfatal heart attacks. This is an ongoing prospective study, which means it is designed to gather data over a specified period of years, involving 120,000 nurses. Other studies conducted in other places throughout the world seem to strongly support the link between estrogen and cardiovascular protection.

Until fairly recently, heart attacks were believed to be a masculine province, caused, some thought, by the excessive stress men endured in the workplace. Heart attacks afflicted men in their forties and fifties while it seemed, women of that age were rarely afflicted. Then medical science found ways to extend both female and male life spans and women began to experience heart attacks in greater numbers and to die from them all too frequently, albeit generally later than men. Researchers began investigating why women in their sixties and early seventies (some ten years later than men) began to experience coronary heart disease (CHD).

29 What protected women prior to this time? Was it estrogen?

Those very questions suggested the need to look into menopause and the estrogen depletion that followed it. At long last, research into CHD and women began in earnest. The results suggested that perhaps estrogen offers protection against the heart attack and stroke-causing blockages that can develop in the blood vessels because it keeps blood vessels flexible by enhancing their elasticity, thus enabling them to function better. Additional studies point to estrogen's positive action upon blood serum lipids, indicating that estrogen increases the high density lipoprotein (HDL), the "good" cholesterol, and decreases the low density lipoprotein (LDL), its "bad" twin. This action enables blood to move smoothly through our blood vessels, which is vital because a heart attack occurs when blood is blocked from reaching the heart. When blood cannot reach the brain, a stroke occurs. Heart disease is the number one killer of American women. In fact, heart attacks and strokes take the lives of more than one million women in the United States and Europe each year.

According to the American Heart Association's *1998 Heart and Stroke Statistical Update*, in terms of total deaths in every year since 1984, coronary vascular disease (CVD) has claimed the lives of more women than men. Even though breast cancer is women's greatest fear and 1 in 26 women will die of breast cancer, the statistic for women dying of CVD is 1 in 2. The total cost of CVD in 1998 is expected to rise to $274.2 billion.

30 What other studies are there concerning women, heart disease, and estrogen?

A number of large-scale studies are under way in the United States and elsewhere in the world. The first major U.S. study to be completed is a three-year, $10 million clinical trial involving more than 850 women under the aegis of the National Institutes of Health (NIH). The results of the Postmenopausal Estrogen-Progestin Intervention (PEPI) trial were released in November 1994 at the American Heart Association's Scientific Sessions. In the PEPI trial, women were divided into five groups. One group took estrogen alone, the second group was given estrogen plus oral micronized progesterone, the third group got estrogen with a synthetic progestin added twelve days per month (the most common HRT regimen), the fourth group got estrogen and progestin continuously all month, and the fifth group received a placebo. Premarin was the estrogen used in the PEPI trial, Provera was the synthetic progestin given, and the oral progesterone was formulated in a laboratory, where it was "micronized," which means it was broken up into tiny particles for better absorption.

Interestingly, the greatest rise in HDL, the "good" cholesterol, was seen in women taking estrogen alone, followed by women taking the natural micronized progesterone with estrogen, who fared better in terms of improvements in lipid levels than women using estrogen and synthetic progestin. The PEPI trial also found that hormone replacement therapy lowers LDL cholesterol and fibrinogen, a blood-clotting factor that is also a predictor of stroke and heart attack. Further, it revealed that none of the treatments in the PEPI trial increased blood pressure, nor did any of the estrogen-progestin combinations cause endometrial hyperplasia (overgrowth of the lining of the uterus, a potentially precancerous condition).

What does all this mean? It means that although some answers have already come from the Nurses' Study and the PEPI trial, there are still holes in the fabric of information concerning estrogen and heart disease. Many more answers will result from the Women's Health Initiative launched by the NIH, which hopes, over a thirteen-year period studying more than 164,500 women at medical centers throughout the United States, to fill in many of the holes. The problem is that we probably can't expect to see the results of that study until 2005 or even later. If you, like me, want and need answers today, we have to work out the risk-to-benefit ratio concerning estrogen and its possible cardiovascular protection for ourselves in partnership with our own physician.

31 Will estrogen help me fight fatigue?

Many studies have shown that estrogen has a mental tonic effect. By that I mean it improves one's mental state, banishes the blues, and, like any good tonic, lifts spirits. In that regard, we might consider estrogen a fatigue fighter, and many women report "just feeling better" once they are taking estrogen. Estrogen can also end those night sweats that disturb sleep, putting an end to insomnia. Even chest palpitations, which always seem worse at night, may disappear with ERT. However, for some women, those with an intact uterus who have to take progesterone as well, that feeling of well-being disappears the minute progesterone is added to their regimen. It is noteworthy that when women switch from synthetic progestin to natural oral micronized progesterone, very frequently the mental tonic effect continues all month undisturbed.

Not to complicate matters further, but when it comes to discussing fatigue, I must mention hypothyroidism (which is discussed in the answer to question 143 in chapter 13) and testosterone replacement therapy. Testosterone, the so-called male hormone, is a great fatigue fighter. I say so-called because what is not discussed as frequently as it should be is the fact that women produce testosterone and that there can be a loss of energy and libido when women lose their testosterone along with their estrogen and progesterone at menopause. Women have 12 to 20 percent of the amount of testosterone men have, but it is that tiny bit of testosterone that spikes our libido and can lift fatigue. In fact, testosterone is the hormone of desire for both men and women, the only hormone that makes us interested in sex.

Doctors have been prescribing a bit of testosterone along with estrogen for women experiencing loss of libido since the late 1960s, with the advent of an oral tablet called Estratest, manufactured by Solvay Pharmaceuticals. Estratest — part estrogen, part testosterone — for many women both lifts flagging libido and fights fatigue. More recently, physicians are offering testosterone by injection (effects last for about a month) and by pellet placed under the skin of the buttocks (effects usually last for three months). These two methods are, of course, more physician-dependent, but work for women for whom Estratest does not. (Testosterone prescriptions can also be filled by compounding pharmacies.) The women whom I interviewed concerning testosterone replacement therapy all indicate that in addition to raising their libido, testosterone helped to get rid of their "menopause headaches" and eliminated their oppressive sense of fatigue.

Most physicians believe that women should not take testosterone without estrogen. As with any good thing, there are drawbacks. The side effects of testosterone replacement therapy may include hirsutism (excessive facial hair), acne, clitoral enlargement or engorgement, and a deepening of the voice. That's why it is so important to seek and work with a physician who is familiar with testosterone replacement for women, who will tailor your prescription to your needs, and who will observe you regularly while you are on the therapy. In the case of the side effects of hirsutism, acne, and enlargement of the clitoris, these conditions will revert to normal once the medication is lessened or stopped completely. Once the voice deepens, however, it stays that way. Most physicians tell me that it is best to start on testosterone replacement very gradually, watching for side effects as you go. That way, you can reap the benefits and negate the side effects.

32 Will estrogen prevent Alzheimer's disease?

Exciting information derived from many clinical studies shows the positive effects of estrogen on mind, mood, and memory. Estrogen's beneficial effects on mental functioning have led to additional important studies indicating that the use of estrogen either reduces the risk of developing Alzheimer's disease or slows the progression of the disease considerably. Early studies done at the University of California at a retirement community, where researchers checked the medical histories of some nine thousand women, found that those on estrogen were 40 percent less likely to develop Alzheimer's disease or other forms of dementia than women who were not on estrogen. Many other studies have seen similar results. Important work has been done by Stanley Birge, M.D., of the division of geriatrics, Washington University School of Medicine, St. Louis, which has demonstrated the valuable effect of estrogen on memory and thinking.

Dr. Barbara Sherwin, professor of psychology and obstetrics and gynecology at McGill University in Montreal, has clearly demonstrated the presence of estrogen receptors on the brain and the effect of lack of estrogen on mind, mood, and memory. A small study done in a Veteran's Administration Hospital in Puget Sound demonstrated that when estrogen was given to Alzheimer's patients, their short-term memory improved. An observational study of 1,124 elderly women in New York City reported in *Lancet* in 1996 suggests that estrogen may lower the risk for Alzheimer's disease by promoting growth of some neurons and stopping accumulation of cerebral amyloid, a substance found in excess in the brains of patients with Alzheimer's.

What does all this mean? As always, it means that more research needs to be done if we can even begin to hope for firm and final answers. It is vital that you understand what Alzheimer's disease is and what it does. Alzheimer's is caused by a loss of brain cells; it is a disease of the nervous system. The disease destroys neurons in parts of the brain involved with cognition — particularly the hippocampus, a structure deep in the brain that plays a role in memory, including the ability to perform familiar tasks. Alzheimer's disease also damages the cerebral cortex, the outer layer of the brain, which is responsible for language and reasoning. Looking at the brain of a patient after autopsy is still the only way physicians can be sure of the diagnosis of Alzheimer's disease. The autopsied brain will invariably show tangles and plaques that have developed among the brain's neurons, along with other physical anomalies.

Named after a German pathologist, Alois Alzheimer, who first identified the disease around the turn of the last century, Alzheimer's disease slowly and unremittingly destroys the mind and the body. Early symptoms of Alzheimer's are the inability to learn or recall information or to find the proper word when speaking, and to become disoriented and when disoriented to become lost. Alzheimer's disease affects an estimated four million Americans annually. By the year 2050 that number is projected to increase to ten million in the United States, where it already ranks among the top ten causes of death.

33 What specific role does estrogen play in preventing Alzheimer's disease?

The eight thousand women enrolled in the Women's Health Initiative Memory Study will help determine what role, if any, ERT plays in preventing this debilitating and devastating disease in women. Preliminary clinical data have shown that the normal loss of estrogen women experience after menopause may be linked to Alzheimer's disease. Evidence has also indicated that the disease may be less likely to strike women who take estrogen after menopause.

The exact mechanism of estrogen's possible effect in the development or progression of Alzheimer's disease is not known. However, research done to date suggests that estrogen works within brain nerve cells (neurons) to ensure the production of enzymes critical to maintaining the connections between the neurons. Specifically, estrogen is thought to make neurons more sensitive to nerve growth factor, a protein that plays a role in the development of axons and dendrites, which transmit and receive messages, respectively, between brain nerve cells. Research has also demonstrated that estrogen increases the production of acetylcholine, one of several brain chemicals that help carry nerve impulses from one neuron to another.

As you read reports of studies concerning estrogen and Alzheimer's disease there are a number of facts you should be aware of. First of all, it is known that Alzheimer's disease is caused partially by some genetic defect, so heredity is a big factor. Alzheimer's disease also strikes women up to three times more often than men. Alzheimer's is most common in individuals over the age of eighty-five, and it might well be that women are more likely to be its victims because, quite simply, women live longer than men. One must also add to the equation the fact that in most of these studies it is likely that healthier and better educated women had chosen to take estrogen, therefore making it unclear to what extent estrogen was responsible for their superior well-being.

Here again, the Women's Health Initiative has launched the first large-scale study concerned with preventing Alzheimer's disease in healthy older women. Bowman Gray School of Medicine in Winston-Salem has taken a leadership role in this endeavor, which will be carried out at forty centers throughout the United States. This WHI study will try to discover whether equilin, a hormone used in Premarin (conjugated equine estrogen), may be the link in stimulating and protecting brain neurons. If so, women might be able to take equilin without running the risk of uterine or breast cancer. Here again, the results are probably at least a decade away.

Some women with a family history of Alzheimer's disease who want to do everything they can to avoid it wonder whether ginkgo biloba works and whether they can take it if they are taking estrogen. I have been taking ginkgo biloba for years along with estrogen. No problem. Call it trying to hedge my bets! For thousands of years, Chinese herbalists have used the leaves of the ginkgo tree to treat memory loss. Now research in the United States suggests that ginkgo may lessen symptoms of Alzheimer's disease. According to the *Encyclopedia of Natural Medicine* by Michael Murray, N.D., and Joseph Pizzorno, N.D., ginkgo biloba has been shown to dilate arteries, veins, and capillaries, thus increasing peripheral circulation and blood flow to the brain. If it does all that, the herb might potentially treat senility, short-term memory loss, and who knows, perhaps other vascular problems. Ginkgo biloba is available over the counter as a capsule or an extract.

34 Will estrogen lower LDL, or "bad" cholesterol?

Studies have shown that estrogen, particularly estrogen taken as an oral tablet, has an impressive impact on the ratio of HDL to LDL cholesterol. This is important because the increase in the good serum cholesterol level works to prevent plaque from clogging our arteries, permitting smoother flow of blood. Estrogen keeps the good cholesterol high and the bad cholesterol low, which helps protect us from coronary heart disease.

35 Will estrogen lift depression?

Yes, if you're asking about the minor depression that can come along as a symptom of menopause. No, if you're speaking of clinical depression. Clinical depression is a debilitating and usually severe condition that can and should be medically treated. Approximately eighteen million Americans suffer from clinical depression, which is often marked by feelings of deep despair, sadness, hopelessness, or anger. This is not the case with post-menopausal blues.

As noted earlier in this chapter, estrogen is the "feel good" hormone, the hormone that can level mood swings, fight nervousness, and help to eliminate anxiety and panic attacks. Many of these are the result of hormonal ups and downs at menopause, and certainly estrogen is a front line contender for ridding ourselves of these conditions.

Studies report that only 25 percent of women encounter minor depression with menopause. From the 25,000 questionnaires I have circulated, that number seems low to me, perhaps because women are not taking into account the anxiety, insomnia, irritability, panic, mood swings, and general nervousness that many of them report under the heading of depression. For women with these symptoms, estrogen may well be the answer.

ERT may lift your spirits, since it modulates the production of serotonin in the brain, and serotonin is the neurotransmitter that gives us that good-to-be-alive feeling. However, for women with an intact uterus, the progestin that they must also take in HRT might well be the hormone of the blues. Recently, studies have noted that women who use oral micronized progesterone, available from compounding pharmacies (see appendix D), instead of the synthetic progestin have far fewer problems with minor depression.

36   Will estrogen reverse my flagging libido?

Estrogen will fight flagging libido only in the sense that it will offer you a mental tonic effect, lifting your spirits and, perhaps, making you more interested in sexual activity because you feel better. Estrogen will also improve lubrication to the vaginal tract, offsetting the thinning and drying that can occur after menopause when your natural estrogen is no longer circulating, thus eliminating painful intercourse, which can be damaging to your libido. Only testosterone is the hormone of desire. If lagging libido is your problem, discuss with your physician the possibility of adding a touch of testosterone to your hormone cocktail. Many women tell me that with the addition of testosterone, their sexual appetite, activity, and satisfaction have improved greatly (but see the answer to question 31 for side effects).

37 Will taking estrogen improve my short-term memory?

Many women are deeply concerned about short-term memory loss: Why can't I remember where I put my sunglasses and car keys? Why can't I remember my thought when I'm in the middle of a sentence? Did I close the garage door before I left home? Did I turn off the oven? What did I come to the grocery store to buy today, anyway? Am I getting old? Am I losing it?

It is frightening, indeed, when memory slips begin to occur, and that fear is understandable. The decline of hormones at menopause can cause short-term memory lapses. Prior to menopause, estrogen works within the synapses and dendrites of the nervous system to permit quick neurotransmission. So before estrogen is lost, there is a rapid ability to recall information and to learn and retain new information. The few studies that have been done have shown that ERT and HRT do make a difference, often returning short-term memory to its premenopausal state. Dr. Barbara Sherwin, an eminent menopause researcher, noted that during the menstrual cycle women experience fluctuating performance of short-term memory. That is probably because estrogen is known to activate the central nervous system, while progesterone may depress it.

We must remember a few other factors. As we age, both men and women may exhibit varying degrees of memory loss. Stress can exacerbate memory loss, create forgetfulness, and dull thinking. Midlife is a stressful time for many women, having nothing to do with menopause; we are often suffering from empty nest syndrome, dealing with the illness and/or death of parents or a spouse, or trying to help with our children's marital and work problems.

So does estrogen help short-term memory loss? Depending on what else is going on in your life, I think by and large it does, and several important studies bear that out. Other studies show that if you wait out those years that surround menopause, the climacteric, memory often returns to its former state intact. Obviously, many more studies need to be done. Perhaps the WHI Memory Study noted in the answer to question 33 will help fill in the blanks.

38 What is the effect of estrogen on osteoarthritis?

Several very recent studies demonstrate a positive effect of estrogen on osteoarthritis. The most significant seems to be the study of more than four thousand Caucasian women over the age of forty-five, reported in the *Archives of Internal Medicine*, 1996, Vol. 156, showing that those women taking estrogen had the lowest incidence of osteoarthritis. This disease, which affects about sixteen million American men and women, can range from uncomfortable to debilitating. It is a completely different disease from osteoporosis. Arthritis is a joint disease and osteoporosis is a bone disease. The most common form of arthritis is osteoarthritis, which is an enlargement, or thickening, of the bones of the joints. Osteoarthritis can be seen most easily in the joints of the fingers, but it is most serious when it involves the knee and hip joints.

People with osteoarthritis typically have very different body types from people with osteoporosis. Individuals with osteoarthritis tend to be larger, in both muscle build and weight. Osteoarthritic growth is usually hard and thick, so people with osteoarthritis of the hips rarely break them. On the other hand, people with osteoporosis are usually smaller, they may be stooped, and their bones, upon observation or testing, are frail and porous. Hip fractures are common in people with osteoporosis. People with osteoarthritis, like people with osteoporosis, still must be concerned with taking appropriate amounts of calcium and exercising regularly.

Then there is rheumatoid arthritis, a crippling disease of the joints. Unlike individuals with osteoarthritis, people with rheumatoid arthritis often have serious problems with osteoporosis. They frequently are sedentary because of painful joints, they often have less calcium circulating in their bloodstream, and they often take cortisone-like drugs, which block calcium absorption into their bones. They have a tendency to break hips and other bones. Rheumatoid arthritis is diagnosed by a blood test.

As usual, more studies need to be done to learn whether estrogen actually does prevent osteoarthritis, but early studies show great promise.

39   Will estrogen protect me from colon cancer?

Colon cancer ranks third after lung and breast cancer as the most common cancer seen in women. Some studies have shown that women on estrogen have appreciably lower rates of colon cancer. In fact, observational studies done fairly recently reported that estrogen lowered women's risk of colon cancer by nearly 50 percent. A study by the American Cancer Society (ACS) agreed with the findings of several smaller studies and found that ERT appears to lower the risk of fatal colon cancer in postmeno-pausal women. The ACS study revealed that women currently using estrogen had a 45 percent reduction in risk when compared to women not using estrogen. The risk reduction grew by another 10 percent for women who had taken estrogen for ten years or longer. That's a 55 percent risk reduction. Conversely, the risk reduction nose-dived to 19 percent for former estrogen users who had stopped.

Much has been written about what is called the "healthy woman effect," meaning that women who take hormones are healthier to begin with, probably get fewer diseases, and get more screening tests, such as the screening test for colon cancer. Like the placebo effect, wherein when you "think" you are taking a medication you feel better, the healthy woman effect is probably real. Yet a risk lowered by 50 percent or more must indicate some benefit from estrogen. Here is an area that is ripe for further research. Current research has shown that estrogen can reduce the bile acids in the colon that can promote tumors, but much more needs to be known.

It is believed that colon cancer begins in the lining of the large intestine in growths called polyps, which then grow to a size that causes bowel obstruction or bleeding or both. Heredity is the largest risk factor for colon cancer, followed by obesity, constipation, and a diet high in red meat. A diet loaded with fiber — fruits, vegetables, and whole grains — can decrease the risk of colon cancer.

40 Can I save my teeth by taking estrogen?

There is a profound relationship between tooth loss and osteoporosis. In fact, osteoporosis may first show up in the mouth. Your dentist may be the first to see a change in bone health, characterized by a change in the strength and density of the jawbones, which hold your teeth in place. Osteoporosis might first be seen as pyorrhea, gum disorders, or any one of the other conditions labeled "periodontal disease." If your teeth seem to be shifting ever so slightly, a bone density test might be in order.

Tooth or gum problems do not necessarily point to osteoporosis, but should be checked out quickly. The fact that periodontal disease is more common in women than in men could lead to the conclusion that the lack of estrogen after menopause has an adverse effect on bone health throughout the body, including the jawbones.

41 Will estrogen eliminate stress incontinence and other bladder problems?

The bladder often reacts negatively to a lack of estrogen after menopause. Common problems include urinary tract infections (UTIs), changes in urgency and frequency in urinating, and stress incontinence. "Among frequent health problems in women, vaginal infections are the ones most likely to be mismanaged," said Dr. Edward Hook III, professor of medicine at the University of Alabama. Vaginal infections often lead to UTIs and bladder problems. For many women estrogen is the answer to bladder problems.

Or UTIs may occur because the tissues of the bladder and the urethra have become thinner and have lost elasticity, and thus are more open to irritation and infection. Since repeated infections can endanger your kidneys and your bladder, see your physician right away.

The frequent need to urinate can be a real pain. As one women said to me recently, "I dare not pass a restroom without stopping in, or I know I'll soon be wet and sorry." Urgency is another problem, and often the urge to urinate is so pronounced that you're concerned that you won't get there in time.

Stress incontinence is thought by many women to be "the worst." It is characterized by leaking a little — or a lot — of urine, when you sneeze, cough, laugh, run after a tennis ball, or otherwise exert yourself. Kegel exercises are very helpful with stress incontinence, but estrogen replacement helps all the above bladder problems if they are caused by a lack of estrogen. Remember the estrogen receptors on the cells that were described earlier? Well, they appear throughout the bladder and the urinary tract. It makes sense that providing them with estrogen again will be helpful.

When it comes to issues of frequency and urgency, often women who have not chosen the estrogen route or who have been told by their physicians that estrogen is not right for them, based on whatever medical condition they might have, develop their own routines, such as making sure they urinate on a regular basis. For example, one woman told me she never lets a full hour go by without urinating.

If stress incontinence is a problem, Kegel exercises are very helpful with bladder control. Kegels also tighten and tone the vaginal area, which can enhance sexual pleasure. Named for Dr. Arnold Kegel, a surgeon at UCLA who developed them in the 1950s, Kegels are easy to do and can be done anywhere without anyone else's being the wiser. There are actually two ways to do Kegels. The first method is to contract your vaginal muscles as if you were trying to hold in your urine. Keep holding in for a count of five, relax for a count of five, and repeat the sequence twenty times. Method two, which seems to work better for some women, is to contract and release the vaginal muscles in quick succession.

Do these twenty times as well. Women often cross-train with Kegel exercises, alternating the two methods. Performing Kegels at least ten times a day can be amazingly helpful. Kegels will not only help you with bladder control but also may keep your pelvic organs functioning well throughout your life. Small effort for a big reward!

42   Will I live longer if I take estrogen?

Who can say? If all the aforementioned benefits of estrogen remain true, and are true for you, you might well live longer. For many women, however, estrogen is their choice for living better for as long as they live. Estrogen perks up our mind, mood, and memory. It plumps up our skin and helps us control our bladder; it makes sexual intercourse more comfortable; it prevents or treats osteoporosis; and it probably protects us against heart disease, stroke, and colon/rectal cancer, and maybe even Alzheimer's disease, osteoarthritis, and other ailments.

When making your personal estrogen decision, you must also consider the risks of estrogen replacement therapy. So read on because these are covered in chapter 4.

4

What Are the Risks of Estrogen Replacement Therapy?

WOMEN talk to other women, and many tell me that they get their best advice and their greatest support from friends and acquaintances who are willing to discuss menopause. We've said it before: Menopause is universal. But how it affects each woman is unique, because each brings to her estrogen decision her own medical history, her own family medical history, and half a lifetime of fears, concerns, and many other deeply personal issues.

What physicians must realize is that each woman will decide for herself whether or not she will take estrogen. She will not be coerced, she will not be threatened, and she will not be cajoled. She also will not be patronized. She will decide.

In order for her to decide, she must have a clear understanding of the risks of estrogen as well as the benefits. She must be able to ask her physician questions and get comprehensible answers, and she must be encouraged to discuss her fears. She needs to know exactly why the physician believes that estrogen is right or wrong for her, whichever the case might be. It's hard to learn all that when her doctor is looking at the watch on the wrist of one hand, while holding the doorknob as if to depart the examination room with the other.

Is it any wonder that patient compliance is the most difficult issue that physicians face? Is it a surprise that most estrogen prescriptions that physicians write are not filled by their confused patients? Is it not understandable that the average length of time most women who do fill their estrogen prescriptions continue to take therapy is only nine months or less?

There are risks, and women have to know about them and be comfortable with them when they start taking estrogen. They have to weigh the risk-to-benefit ratio for themselves carefully and balance the scales in their own favor.

When we consider risks, it is important to remember that the first negative reports about estrogen therapy came to light around 1976. That's when studies demonstrated a link between estrogen replacement therapy and endometrial cancer (cancer of the lining of the uterus) in postmenopausal women. Every day since then there has been an uphill battle as we women try to overcome our worst nightmares, those of agreeing to take estrogen when it might cause us serious health problems later in our lives. That fear flies in the face of many studies that show benefit after benefit for estrogen therapy. No one should simply dismiss our fears. We have to deal with them. Let's take the toughest, most confusing question first.

43 Does estrogen cause cancer?

It is known that estradiol is the most potent form of estrogen in the body. It is also known that when there is too much estradiol in the body or it is there for too long, it can cause problems. You will recall that when estrogen was used alone in the years following publication of Dr. Wilson's book, cases of uterine cancer were reported and doctors stopped prescribing it. So for the most part estrogen wasn't in much demand until it was determined that cycling it with progestin would protect the uterus while offering the benefits of estrogen to the rest of the body. Research studies had already suggested that estrogen, when unopposed by progestin, might prove carcinogenic to estrogen-sensitive tissues such as those in the uterus.

It is known that estrogen should be used cautiously, if at

all, by women with a strong history of cancer of the endometrium or of estrogen-dependent breast cancer. It is important to note that in each case, estrogen does not cause cancer. In terms of endometrial cancer, estrogen can cause the lining of the uterus (the endometrium) to build up, causing endometrial hyperplasia, a precancerous condition, if it is used without some form of progesterone.

44 Isn't breast cancer every woman's number one concern?

Yes, breast cancer is the main fearful issue that women deal with, and numerous studies indicate it to be their number one concern, particularly when it is estimated that one out of nine women will, at sometime during her lifetime, develop breast cancer. That statistic is so frightening that women have told me they have literally looked around an auditorium filled with women and then down their particular row and have begun counting off: "One, two, three, four — oh God, don't let number nine be me!" Irrational fear, you say. No way. It's there, and we must respond to it with reason and unvarnished facts. We need facts from significant studies that have not been massaged and altered to fit into one expert or another's point of view or argument.

A 1997 report of a survey of more than a thousand women between the ages of forty-five and sixty-four by the National Council on the Aging (NCOA), entitled "Myths and Misperceptions About Aging and Women's Health," revealed that women are misinformed about their risks of some age-related diseases, such as heart disease and cancer. When asked which disease they fear the most, 61 percent of the women surveyed said cancer. Only 9 percent said heart attack, which is the number one killer of women. Furthermore, the women surveyed were not aware that since 1987 lung cancer has claimed more women's lives than breast cancer. The confusion can be deadly, because it may deter women from making appropriate decisions regarding their postmenopausal health.

To add to the misperceptions, a case study by Vincent T. Covello, Ph.D., director of the Center for Risk Communications in New York City, designed to determine women's perceptions of the risks of age-related diseases, including breast cancer, found that most of the women surveyed believed incorrectly that lifetime statistics about the risk of diseases such as breast cancer applied to their own age groups. One of the consequences of this perception, as it relates to breast cancer, is that fear of the disease may result in overlooking or disregarding important therapies such as HRT or ERT.

The truth is that *one woman in nine over the course of her lifetime* encounters that level of risk. At age fifty-one, the average age for menopause, our risk is more likely to be one woman out of fifty. Actually, the indications are fairly straightforward when it comes to estrogen and breast cancer. Women who have had estrogen-dependent breast cancer will usually not be given estrogen. (I say usually, because as I travel the country and interview physicians, I have learned that some will offer short-term, carefully-monitored estrogen to women who have had breast cancer in the past but whose menopausal symptoms are so debilitating that they have difficulty functioning.)

It is important to know that estrogen does not cause cancer and that estrogen is not a carcinogen, but it can stimulate the growth of cancer that is already in place. There are two primary physician concerns at work here. One is the fear of exposing the patient with a strong family history of breast cancer to the risk, and the other is worrying that estrogen might cause a recurrence of the disease in a woman who has already had breast cancer.

45 Are all breast cancers estrogen-dependent?

No. Yet women often ignore or are unaware of this. Not surprisingly, some studies show that estrogen-dependent breast cancer is more common in younger women, who are still in the reproductive stage of their lives, and fairly uncommon in women who are several years beyond menopause. Non-estrogen-dependent breast cancer is more common among postmenopausal women. Tests can determine whether or not a breast cancer is estrogen-dependent.

But what about me, and women like me, who have not had breast cancer and do not have the disease in their families? I'm told the indications for us are not at all clear-cut. One study has shown that for women between age sixty and sixty-six, using estrogen increases their risk significantly. Another group of studies demonstrates the impact of exposure to certain pesticides as the culprits causing breast cancer, because once in the body these pesticides are said to mimic the actions of estrogen. Yet a study reported by Harvard researchers in the September 19, 1997, issue of the *Journal of the National Cancer Institute* concerning regional breast cancer differences found that not to be so. Statistics show that more women die of breast cancer in the northeastern United States than in the South and that the rates for the Midwest and West lie somewhere in between. However, when breast cancer risk factors were taken into account, social and lifestyle forces rather than local environmental pollutants appeared to play a role in a woman's susceptibility. Many studies show no increase in risk of breast cancer to women on estrogen, while others do show a correlation between estrogen therapy and breast cancer!

Overall, however, the data seems to suggest, and many menopause experts seem to believe, that taking estrogen short-term does not increase the risk of breast cancer. When I attended a meeting of the International Menopause Society in Stockholm a few years ago, the consensus seemed to be that women were safe on estrogen for perhaps ten to fifteen years, after which the risk of breast cancer increased by 20 to 30 percent.

46 How can I get a handle on this confusing breast cancer/ estrogen stuff?

It has to be put into perspective. First, there are risk factors to consider, such as early onset of menstruation, late menopause, and never having been pregnant. These are considered possible risk factors because they indicate a long and uninterrupted period of time during which the body is exposed to its own natural estrogen. There are also lifestyle risk factors like eating a high-fat diet and drinking more than one ounce of alcohol, four ounces of wine, or twelve ounces of beer per day that have to be factored into the equation, because these have been shown to increase risk. A study that included more than 300,000 women demonstrated that among women who averaged less than one drink a day, the breast cancer risk was 9 percent higher than teetotalers. Among women who reported having two to five drinks a day, breast cancer risk rose by 41 percent.

Activity and lifestyle choices should enter into your personal equation. Do you practice breast self-examination monthly? Do you see your physician at least once a year, and is a manual breast exam performed during that visit? Do you have an annual mammogram? These are all proven methods of detecting breast cancer, and breast cancer when found early is often curable. Oh, and that's another important point to add to your equation: if, for example, there is a cancer growing slowly and silently in your breast and it is estrogen-dependent, and estrogen replacement therapy causes it to grow faster and be found sooner and removed, mightn't you be better off in the long run? That's really the big question when it comes to estrogen and breast cancer. Think about it.

47 What do the studies show concerning elevation in breast cancer risk from taking estrogen?

The studies and meta analysis (that is, the study of a group of studies) all differ somewhat on this point. Current research gives no definite answers and offers no clear path to an answer. It doesn't indicate that the use of the right dose of estrogen has significantly elevated the risk or added to the number of breast cancer cases in the United States. Yes, some studies have indicated that long-term estrogen takers have a slight increase in breast cancer risk. According to Dr. Isaac Shiff, writing in his book *Menopause*, some postmenopausal women over the age of fifty who have been on estrogen replacement therapy for seven to ten years do show a distinct risk of breast cancer compared with women not using ERT or HRT.

Research does show that estrogen can adversely affect breast tissue for some women over time. The dose of estrogen coupled with the length of time you take it seems to affect risk. Whether you are on ERT or HRT seems to be important. The confounding fact here is that the American Cancer Society reports that the incidence of breast cancer has stopped escalating since 1987, even though the use of HRT and ERT has grown. So far, the connections between breast cancer risk and estrogen remain ill-defined, but they are there. So decisions become a woman's choice and should be dependent on all the risk factors — family and personal medical history, symptoms, and quality-of-life issues, as well as fear and other concerns.

A genetic defect in the genes, known as BRCA1 and BRCA2, must also be taken into consideration. Three studies in the *New England Journal of Medicine*, May 15, 1997, help to clarify the risk, but they noted that these damaged genes are not the sole determinants of cancer risk. A genetic mutation does not guarantee cancer. An earlier study, reported in the *New England Journal of Medicine (NEJM)*, April 17, 1997, reinforced limited screening of high-risk women, because it is not clear that women would benefit from having BRCA1 or BRCA2 identified.

It is fairly clear that women need to continue to do breast self-examination and to make sure they are doing it correctly, see their physician at least yearly for a manual breast exam, and have regular mammograms. A study reported in *Cancer*, August 15, 1997, suggests that women perform breast self-exams monthly and have their annual mammogram done right after a menstrual period.

In the meantime, there is still no agreement on how early in life mammograms should start, and the NIH consensus panel recommends that women make individual decisions. So the tug-of-war between starting mammography at age forty or not beginning until age fifty remains at a stalemate. According to the *Journal of the National Cancer Institute*, April 16, 1997, the United States is not alone in recommending mammography screening for women ages forty to forty-nine but clearly doesn't have much company worldwide. Of the twenty-one countries surveyed by the International Breast Cancer Screening Database Council, only Iceland, Sweden, and one province in Canada also recommended screening for women in their forties.

48 Can a postmenopausal woman on estrogen replacement therapy become pregnant?

Usually not. ERT is typically prescribed after the ovaries have run out of eggs and the estrogen that they produced has diminished and then disappeared. So, no eggs, no pregnancy. But what if, for example, a woman hasn't had a period for four or five months and figures she's in the clear? And then her ovaries turn on one more time, produce an egg that meets the sperm coming the other way, and conception takes place? Pregnancy occurs.

That possibility is why physicians up until just a few years ago suggested that women switch from birth control pills to another form of contraception after the age of forty-five and that they wait one full year without a period before considering themselves "safe" from pregnancy. Another contributing factor was that neither the serum estradiol concentration nor FSH blood tests are reliable indicators of reduced estrogen production if a woman is on oral contraceptives, which, of course, do contain estrogen, until she switches to HRT or ERT. Today many physicians tell women that they can guide them from perimenopause to menopause with no symptoms, using low-dose birth control pills, which also do contain estrogen, which is just great.

A surprise pregnancy doesn't often occur but it could, and it is a good idea to use contraception until at least one year after what you believe to have been your final period.

49 I have a uterine fibroid tumor. Can I take estrogen?

Many women with fibroid tumors want to know if they can even consider taking estrogen. The medical answer to that question was formerly a fairly universal no, but today's low-dose estrogen prescriptions may change that answer to a "maybe, let's try it" for some women. Although the answer to the questions about fibroid tumors is often a conundrum, for many women the situation plays out like this: A woman, I'll call her Alexa, has a large estrogen-receptive fibroid tumor. When it caused problems and pain, her physician had on many occasions suggested a hysterectomy, removing her uterus and the offending fibroid. The only alternative he could offer was for her to wait for menopause, at which time the tumor, no longer being fed estrogen, would undoubtedly shrink. Alexa chose the second alternative and waited out the discomfort caused by the fibroid. Her menopausal process began, and she had a terrible time. She was hot, sleepless, and nasty, by her own description.

When she made the decision to wait, she hadn't added into the equation the fact that her menopausal symptoms might be so bad as to greatly diminish the otherwise good quality of her life. She went back to her physician. He again offered her a hysterectomy. "No way," she said. "I toughed it out this long, I'm not going to consider surgery now." Alexa thought it was time to get another opinion, so she consulted another gynecologist.

After reviewing her long and involved history with her fibroid, her new doctor told her that sometimes, carefully monitored low-dose estrogen replacement could be offered short-term to women with a fibroid tumor. Alexa was overjoyed. She has been on estrogen now for over a year. Her menopausal symptoms have vanished, and interestingly enough, the estrogen has not stimulated growth of the fibroid. That may not be the outcome for other cases, but it is one that you should know about, so that if you are having a similar problem you can discuss with your physician whether you can consider estrogen. An interesting bit of research showed that women using transdermal estrogen therapy (patches) plus a progestin had an increase in the growth of fibroids, but that women taking both estrogen and progestin in tablet form did not. Many of the contraindications for taking estrogen have changed since additional research has been done and there are some new answers to old questions.

These questions do need to be answered when you consider that fibroids, outgrowths of the uterus, are very common. Nearly one-third of women have them by the time they reach menopause. Most of the time they can be ignored, unless of course they cause problems, such as bleeding or other symptoms like digestive or bladder complications, because of their size. There is a fairly new surgical procedure called a myomectomy, during which fibroids are removed from the uterus through the vagina or through an abdominal incision, leaving the uterus intact. This works only for women who have just a few fibroids, and sometimes, because of the normal estrogen circulating in your body continuing to feed them, they do regrow, necessitating another procedure. Myomectomy is not a full or final answer to fibroids, but it is one about which you should be aware.

50   I have had phlebitis. Can I consider ERT?

Phlebitis is a circulatory problem in which a vein becomes inflamed. In the past, circulatory and vascular problems usually precluded a woman's using estrogen. These days the scientific community is divided on that point. I interviewed a number of physicians who believe that some form of estrogen can be prescribed for women with phlebitis, if the patient is carefully and frequently monitored. You should be aware that in the fall of 1996 three studies were reported that showed a double or quadruple increase in phlebitis in the legs of women taking estrogen and that those numbers prevailed no matter whether a woman was on estrogen alone or estrogen and progestin. Furthermore, some physicians still rule estrogen out if a woman has experienced any clotting problems, such as thrombophlebitis. Others will make an exception for one such instance, but believe repeated episodes of phlebitis or other clotting problems make estrogen a bad choice.

While we're discussing phlebitis, we should also delve into other circulatory problems that represent a contraindication to ERT. These problems fall under the heading of thromboembolic disease, in which the body forms blood clots. This includes clots in the veins (thrombophlebitis), clots in the lungs (pulmonary emboli), and clots in the arteries of the legs. A heart attack or stroke caused by a blood clot having traveled and then blocked an artery in either the heart or the carotid artery to the brain is also considered thromboembolic. There is some concern that estrogen may increase clotting, that the higher the dose the greater the risk. The risk escalates for women who smoke, because smoking increases the risk of circulatory and vascular problems. There are other studies that don't find that effect.

So what's the definitive answer? Unfortunately, there is none. If you have circulatory problems and take estrogen, you're taking a gamble.

51 Will I gain weight if I take estrogen?

I repeat: estrogen does not significantly increase your weight! However, many women that I have interviewed insist that estrogen makes them hungrier (perhaps because it makes them feel better, so they are more active). Approximately one in four women report a slight weight gain after starting on estrogen therapy. Whether this is actually fatty tissue or water retention is not clear, but the problem persists. It shows on the scale. It also shows in the way our clothes fit, or cease to fit.

This problem may be more one of timing than of medication, because menopause typically occurs when our metabolism has shifted to low gear. That shift may be the culprit. As if that weren't enough, the number of calories we women need decreases between 2 and 8 percent for every decade after our twentieth birthday. Let's figure this out: Say you're fifty today and your caloric age-influenced reduction was somewhere in the middle — say, about 5 percent. Well, you're three decades past twenty, so you probably require 15 percent fewer calories at this age. Obviously, how and what you consume and how much you exercise will affect this percentage greatly.

Now take into consideration that as we age our percentage of lean muscle mass declines while our percentage of body fat increases. What does that tell us? It again points to the fact that keeping weight off depends on sensible nutrition and a regular exercise regimen. Before we get into healthful nutrition and determining the best exercise program, let's return to the metabolic burn. Statistics from the field of nutrition inform us that from about the age of thirty-five on, our metabolism slows between ½ and 1 percent per year. So again, let's say you are fifty and your metabolism is one of those 1 percent per year slow-downers. Well, by your current age, your metabolism has probably slowed by 15 percent. So anyway you figure, there is a 15 percent slowdown. Now, looking at the ranges we've discussed, you can recognize the spectrum of individual differences. If you are lucky your metabolism has slowed only by 7½ percent or so, but even then you've got to make up for the change if staying at your same weight is your ultimate goal. And that is an excellent goal in terms of your good health.

52 What can women do to avoid gaining weight after menopause and while taking estrogen?

What is a good diet for this time of life? That's another question I receive often from my readers. The simplest answer is that what we should eat at this time of life is probably the same kind of healthful food that we should have eaten throughout our life. Most experts are quick to point out that eating right greatly influences our continued good health and our energy quotient. Our diet should be guided by the need to lower fat, increase fiber, and pack in calcium-rich foods. Women tell me they have tried every crash diet that has been popularized, and their weight has yo-yo'd for so many years that it gets harder and harder to lose weight. That's because typically with every quick-fix diet, you lose fat and muscle, and with each return of the weight you get back more fat. Since lean muscle tissue enables us to burn fat more efficiently, our bodies' ability to use calories wisely is compromised each time we do the dieting ups-and-downs.

The main thrust of reducing fat in the body should be to reduce fat intake. That's because fat makes fat, which plants itself quickly on our hips and thighs, creating the apple shape that we're told is predictive of heart disease. Try to keep your fat intake between 20 and 30 grams per day. Remember that protein and carbohydrates are good choices, since they contain less than half the calories of fat. The healthiest diet is made up largely of vegetables, fruits, and whole grains.

Don't forget to couple your sensible reduced-fat eating with a good exercise plan that contains the three kinds of exercise we women need: stretching for flexibility, aerobic exercise to protect our hearts, and weight-bearing exercise to protect our bones. The number one weight-bearing exercise is walking, according to a National Sporting Goods Association survey, so a daily five-minute stretch followed by twenty to thirty minutes of brisk walking and a five-minute stretching cool-down is really all you need to do. Resistance training with weights also adds to total body fitness, keeping our muscles strong and maintaining the mineral density of our bones to keep osteoporosis at bay. Resistance training results in increased muscle mass, and extra muscle speeds up metabolism, enabling us to burn more calories. The American College of Sports Medicine recommends that healthy adults work out with weights twice each week if they have no medical condition that precludes resistance training. If you are not sure, check with your doctor. If weight workouts are okay for you, learn how to use weights properly from a trainer. Learn more about midlife nutrition and exercise in chapter 11.

53 My mother and sister have had breast cancer. Can I take estrogen?

Women with your family history are rightfully concerned about using estrogen. Most women in your situation don't want to take estrogen, and most physicians do not want to prescribe it for them. Studies done by the National Institutes of Health have shown that the risk of breast cancer is double for a woman who has a sister or a mother who has had breast cancer. Typically, if the mother's breast cancer appeared in the years before she experienced menopause, the daughter's risk is even higher. Considering estrogen then becomes a real high-wire act, and other health issues come into play. For example, if your menopause symptoms are debilitating, some physicians will consider short-term, frequently monitored ERT. If your family history also contains risk factors for osteoporosis, heart disease, or Alzheimer's disease as well as for breast cancer, a decision in favor of estrogen may be made considering these statistics: nine times more women die of heart disease than breast cancer; osteoporosis is the fourth leading killer of women; and protection from or slowing down Alzheimer's disease with estrogen replacement has shown great promise in numerous studies.

The answer to your question just got easier with the FDA's approval of Evista, the exciting "designer estrogen" mentioned earlier and which will be discussed more thoroughly in chapter 8. Osteoporosis treatment medications that already have FDA approval, such as Fosamax and Miacalcin, are discussed in detail in chapter 3.

54 Does high blood pressure interfere with my ability to take estrogen?

The Menopause Time of Life, a 1986 publication of the U.S. Department of Health and Human Services, lists high blood pressure (hypertension) among the conditions that preclude women's using estrogen. Conversely, data from the recent PEPI study (see question 30 in chapter 3) demonstrate that estrogen, taken either alone or along with progestin for women with an intact uterus, does not seem to raise blood pressure, at least not within the three-year period of the study. Newer findings actually suggest that women who have had high blood pressure in the past might benefit from estrogen, since estrogen may reduce the incidence of stroke and heart attack. If you and your doctor considered and ruled out estrogen in the past because of high blood pressure, you may want to revisit the subject.

Estrogen delivered by transdermal therapy (the patch, discussed in chapter 5), which enables the estrogen to bypass the liver, the kidneys, and the digestive system initially, was a possibility for women with certain kinds of hypertension even before the PEPI study began. That is because estrogen taken by patch or via vaginal cream (see question 63) did not seem to affect blood pressure, possibly because it does not cause the release of enzymes (renin and angiotensin) from the kidneys, which, in turn, can raise blood pressure, as it does in about five women out of a hundred who take estrogen by mouth.

If you experience an increase in your blood pressure very shortly after taking estrogen tablets, then estrogen taken orally is not for you. Your physician will probably suggest that you switch to the patch. Most physicians seem to agree that women with high blood pressure can use some form of estrogen that will not affect blood pressure. Often it is a matter of watching closely and being prepared and amenable to switching products. Since high blood pressure can lead to heart attack and stroke, having your blood pressure checked regularly is important, whether or not you choose to take estrogen. Remember, hypertension is called the silent killer because no symptoms herald its presence. One of the best ways to reduce blood pressure is to lose weight.

55   I had a heart attack when I was forty-seven. I'm now fifty-five. Can I take estrogen?

Many studies have shown that when women with a history of heart disease take estrogen, they may have less chance of recurrent heart problems and better chances of living longer. See the answers to Questions 56 and 80 for newer, though not conclusive, information. Some reports demonstrate that there is a very high percentage (between 70 and 90 percent) reduction in mortality for women with heart disease who begin to take estrogen; others disagree.

This might have to do with the fact that when estrogen is used as a preventive against heart disease in otherwise healthy women, a reduction in cholesterol is noted. When, however, estrogen is provided to women with heart disease, it additionally seems to elevate the functioning and increase the elasticity of the blood vessels. Having had a heart attack at the age of forty-seven certainly places you at the younger end of the scale, since most women do not suffer coronary heart disease or heart attacks prior to menopause.

It is during the decade after our menopause that we women

begin to catch up to men in regard to heart disease. Our ten-year grace period vis-à-vis heart disease probably exists because we have had estrogen in our bodies until the age of menopause. It appears that our own natural estrogen protected our hearts by raising the level of HDL cholesterol, the good stuff, which sweeps through our arteries, removing plaque and keeping those fatty substances from sticking to artery walls.

56 What significant studies have been done concerning estrogen and heart disease?

The long-term Nurses' Health Study, begun in 1976, indicated a close association between estrogen deficiency and heart disease risk. The three-year, $3 million PEPI trial, funded primarily by the National Heart, Lung, and Blood Institute of the National Institutes of Health, was the first major study to research the effects of hormone replacement therapy and estrogen replacement therapy on menopausal women and provided some interesting information in regard to women and heart disease. It showed hormone replacement therapy's positive impact on blood cholesterol. Because the study was short-term, it was not possible to draw definitive conclusions about its long-term benefit to cardiovascular health. It did, however, reveal that estrogen not only protects against bone loss but also increases bone mineral density in the spine and hips.

A report from the Heart and Estrogen-Progestin Replacement Study (HERS), a five-year, $40 million study designed to examine whether HRT will reduce the frequency of new cardiovascular disease incidents in women with preexisting cardiovascular disease illuminated some of the short-term effects of combined estrogen and progestin on heart disease. More than two thousand postmenopausal women with coronary heart disease were recruited for this study. Results were reported in the *Journal of the American Medical Association* (August 19, 1998) and cast doubt on the broadly held medical belief that women who already have heart disease can benefit from HRT after menopause. (See Question 80.) And, of course, look for information from the mother of all women's health studies, the NIH Women's Health Initiative (WHI) involving more than 164,500 women over a period of thirteen years. It is unfortunate that its data won't be available until 2005, for it may provide us with a lot of important information many of us would like to have now. The WHI was designed to study the effects of hormone therapy on heart disease, breast cancer, and osteoporosis. Whatever the findings turn out to be, it does appear that estrogen has therapeutic value to the circulatory system.

57   I have diabetes. Can I take estrogen?

You probably can and should take estrogen. The estrogen used in replacement therapy is usually of such low doses that it can be used by women with diabetes. That is because estrogen rarely affects the metabolism of sugar. If you and your physician decide that estrogen might be good for you, she or he will probably want to monitor your blood sugar levels fairly frequently.

As you know all too well, diabetes is a disease caused by a problem with metabolizing sugar. Juvenile diabetes (now referred to as insulin-dependent diabetes) usually occurs, as the name implies, in childhood. It occurs because of the body's failure to produce sufficient insulin, and daily insulin injections are usually necessary to compensate for this failure. The second type of diabetes is much more common and often appears in postmenopausal women. It is called adult-onset diabetes or non–insulin dependent diabetes. The difference between type I and type II very simply is that in adult-onset diabetes the body does make insulin, but for unknown reasons it is unable to use it.

The hereditary factor, obesity, and high blood pressure often set the stage for adult-onset diabetes, which may develop in women after menopause. Weight loss and exercise frequently can control diabetes. If diabetes remains uncontrolled, either type I or type II, the stage is set for coronary heart disease. Diabetes has a deleterious effect on the tiny arteries throughout the body, and when you couple diabetes with high blood pressure, obesity, high cholesterol, and high triglycerides, you are setting the stage for a fourfold increased risk of heart disease. When it comes to heart attack, this is a significant survival problem for women in general, and for the diabetic woman in particular. The bottom line appears to indicate that estrogen can be your ally in your long-term battle against CHD.

58 If I take estrogen will I go on menstruating forever?

Forever is a long time. Today there are ways to take estrogen that may help you enjoy its benefits while getting rid of your monthly periods. First let's look at exactly why you continue menstruating. You will recall that in the introduction we discussed how each month an egg is released from one of your ovaries, and that signals your estrogen and progesterone production plant to get to work. The estrogen and progesterone prepare the lining of the uterus to accept a fertilized egg. When no fertilized egg takes hold, the lining is shed in menstruation and the cycle begins anew.

That can be likened to hormone replacement therapy in the following way: You take estrogen from day 1 to day 25 of the month, add progestin for the last 12 or 13 days that you are taking estrogen, and then stop taking both hormones for the rest of the month. What occurs is that the lining of your uterus sloughs off and you menstruate, in what is called withdrawal bleeding. But today there is a new way to take estrogen and progesterone, in what has been named continuous combined therapy. With this regimen, you take both estrogen and usually a lower dose of progestin every day of the month, every day of the year. This type of therapy should end the problem of menstruating in anywhere from three to six months. It can be a boon as well because the lower dose of progestin often eliminates those dreadful PMS-like symptoms. There is an interesting theory behind the continuous combined approach, and that is that the hormone receptors in the uterus, being bombarded by hormones daily, eventually become exhausted and the uterine lining stops growing altogether. (Of course, none of this pertains to women who have had a hysterectomy, who, if they do choose to take estrogen, can take it without progestin.)

If you want to try the continuous combined approach for long-term benefits, be prepared for a rocky road of irregular bleeding in the early months. Older women frequently have fewer problems with this regimen, because they might bleed less, simply because their uterine lining may be less responsive to the hormones.

There are new products for both the sequential therapy and the continuous combined therapy, Premphase and Prempro respectively. They will be covered in detail in Question 88.

59   I tried oral estrogen, had a gallbladder attack, and quit. Can I consider estrogen again and manage to avoid gallbladder problems?

A dear friend of mine was carried off a plane in excruciating pain. When she was finally made comfortable in the hospital, her diagnosis came back — she had passed a stone. She never had gallbladder disease and immediately suspected estrogen, the only new addition to her lifestyle. She quit taking estrogen because, as she said, "I never want that kind of pain again." Now, with the newest studies showing that estrogen protects us from so many diseases, she is rethinking her decision. That's probably wise.

Let's take a moment to discuss the relationship between estrogen and gallbladder disease. Changes in estrogen levels affect how bile in the body is metabolized. Those changes can result in gallstone formation. Because of the impact of estrogen, gallbladder disease is more common in women. Some studies have shown that women taking oral tablets such as Premarin have a greater risk of gallbladder complications. The studies indicate that the risk is higher if you are currently on the hormone and that it dramatically decreases about five years after you stop. So, if that is the case, my friend is right in her decision.

That may be so with oral estrogen, but what about the

patch, cream, or the newest contender, the vaginally-placed estrogen ring, a product of Pharmacia & Upjohn named Estring, all of which may not carry the risk of gallbladder problems. In the case of the patch, that may be because the estrogen delivered transdermally (through the skin) initially bypasses the liver.

Gallstones, although rarely fatal, can be extremely painful. Sometimes surgery is indicated, and it comes with its own bag of risks and benefits. So what is my friend to do? She knows that the risk factors for gallbladder disease include a high-fat diet, obesity, and a family history of gallbladder disease. Interestingly, she has none of these. She has been resting her estrogen decision on that one gallstone attack, which she claims was enough to last a lifetime. Yet she is reopening her estrogen file and will look at it afresh, considering all the new information.

60 Can a woman consider estrogen after she has had endometrial cancer?

That is another former no-no that is being reevaluated and reconsidered. Conventional thinking has long held that ERT after endometrial cancer was not a good idea, because more than 80 percent of endometrial cancers are estrogen-dependent. Two studies in the late 1980s, however, suggested that estrogen replacement therapy does not increase the risk of recurrence.

In an attempt to clarify this issue, a large new study will compare estrogen replacement therapy to a placebo in more than two thousand women who have had surgery for early-stage endometrial cancer. Women in the study in both groups will have checkups every six months for three years and then annually for two more years. Here again, it will be several years before any results are available, and, as we know, they may not provide the final answer. This is an area of concern that you will want to discuss with your own physician. Talk about Evista, the newly FDA approved SERM (selective estrogen receptor modulator), which is blocked out of the tissues of the uterus and breast yet mimics estrogen in some other parts of the body.

61 I've had breast cancer, but my menopause symptoms are making me miserable and nonfunctional. Can I take ERT at all?

This chapter began with a discussion of breast cancer. It is appropriate that it close with it as well. The breast cancer questions continue unabated, because breast cancer continues to loom as women's greatest fear, even though heart disease is our number one killer. As explained earlier, some physicians will consider short-term, carefully monitored estrogen replacement therapy for women who have had breast cancer and whose menopause symptoms are debilitating. It is a tough call.

Make sure you are in a comfortable patient-physician partnership, then sit down with your doctor and review the risks and benefits of the estrogen course of action. If you have risk factors for other diseases — heart disease and osteoporosis, for example — add that information to your equation. You can discuss Evista, the new estrogen compound that eliminates risk to breast and uterine tissue but offers protection to bone and heart. If there are lifestyle changes you haven't yet made, such as improving your diet and exercising more, throw that into the discussion as well. Talk about alternative methods of therapy that can alleviate your menopause symptoms — from acupuncture to visualization. Look into herbal and vitamin choices, which may work (they are covered in chapter 10). Put all this information together with the key piece, which is whether or not your breast cancer was estrogen-dependent, and make your decision with your doctor's guidance.

Estrogen — The Pharmaceuticals

5

What Estrogen Products Are Available?

WHEN it comes to taking estrogen, the major problem to-day is confusion. There are more products than women can even imagine and new ones keep entering the pipe-line. The formulas for these products are often quite dif-ferent from one another. That's both good and bad news. Good, because it means that if one product doesn't work well for you, you can try another. Bad news, because, according to Elizabeth Barrett-Connor, M.D., one of the pioneers in research-ing women's postmenopausal health, physicians often stay with their own prescribing practices. By this Dr. Barrett-Connor means that they continue to prescribe for 90 percent of their patients what they've always prescribed, instead of tailoring the estrogen product to the patient. So a doctor who has always prescribed Premarin, which has been the gold standard of estrogen since the 1940s, will continue to prescribe it. It is up to the patient to come back and say "This doesn't work for me, for these reasons. Can we try something else?"

Unfortunately, many women don't know that other prod-ucts may affect them quite differently and thus don't play out that scenario. Instead they just stop taking their estrogen, don't bother to taper off, as suggested in chapter 2, and don't bother to let their physicians know until their next visit that they have discontinued therapy. Or wary women, feeling unsure and not fully informed, never fill the prescription given them in the first place. Some women have told me they carried their estrogen prescriptions around in their purses for a long while, and when finally the bits of paper became flimsy and fuzzy, like purse lint, they opted not to take them to their pharmacists. Sooner or later the prescription simply disappeared.

Patient compliance is often acknowledged to be the practicing physician's number one problem. I hate the word and the idea of compliance. It sounds so militaristic. I would sooner say that the patient is not living up to her end of the bargain in the patient-physician partnership. But is the physician? And was the partnership carefully structured and fully acknowledged and agreed to by both parties? Without agreement between the physician and the patient to work together in the best interests of the patient's health and well-being, there is no possibility of achieving a comfortable working relationship. How then can the lines of communication remain open and the physician provide and the patient benefit from the best possible health care?

The advent of managed care has made an already bad patient-care situation even worse. Since the health care delivery system is now at its worst, women must be at their best, pursuing excellent health and health care with dogged determination and armed with abundant information. I believe that the baby boomers may still be able to cut through the paperwork maze of a depersonalized system and that all women will ultimately benefit from their pioneering spirit. That's what that large group of people born between 1946 and 1964 is recognized for — challenging the status quo. The question remains and is begging for an answer: Will the baby boomers also significantly change health care as it is provided to menopausal and postmenopausal women? I hope so.

Beginning in January 1996, the leading edge of the baby boomers started celebrating their big Five-Oh. Fifty, as you already know, for the women in that group spells menopause. Consider the fact that each day since that fateful January, another

3,500 to 4,000 baby boomer women enter the menopausal age range. Some see this as the marketing opportunity of a lifetime for companies that produce estrogen products. I don't see it that way. I see it as a marketing obligation that should have three major thrusts. First, women must be better informed about the risks and benefits of estrogen replacement therapy. Second, physicians must be better informed about the real needs and concerns of women and must respond to them in a vastly improved, more timely manner. Last, both physicians and their patients must learn about tailoring the prescription to the individual. This just isn't happening, and hormone replacement therapy, instead of being customized, is offered initially as a one-size-fits-all solution.

I can tell you from my lecturing travels that women simply are not informed about how many different estrogen products and strengths, or dosages, are available. They are also not aware of the different methods, or regimens, by which they can take estrogen. Women frequently read about the arguments concerning whether menopause has been medicalized (whatever that means) and whether menopause is an "estrogen-deficiency disease" or a "natural transition." Women tell me that they are not interested in those deliberations, preferring instead solid information that enables them to choose what they wish to do about short-term relief of the nuisance symptoms of menopause as well as long-term preventive therapy. Women simply want to feel better and get on with their lives.

Occasionally those kinds of arguments end up in print, doing women more harm than good. Watching Dr. Susan Love, a breast surgeon, on television promoting her hormone book and constructing a conspiracy between the pharmaceutical companies that manufacture estrogen products and some physicians is a case in point. That kind of talk undermines the physician-patient relationship. Giving her the benefit of the doubt, I wonder whether she is a single-focused humanitarian looking only at women as breasts, forgetting the other parts of our bodies that estrogen protects?

In the June 9, 1997, issue of *The New Yorker*, writer Malcolm Gladwell took Dr. Love and her hormone book to task, faulting her for her prejudicial stand. He wrote, "What Love has done is recalculate the risk/benefit equation for estrogen, which is fine, except she consistently overstates the risks and understates the benefits." He continued, "Incredibly, however, Love has her numbers backward: in women younger than seventy-five, there are actually more than three times as many deaths from heart disease as from breast cancer." It's hard to know what to make of this kind of error.

Another thing that concerns me is why women have gone on so long in their supplicant roles when it comes to health care. The why probably is connected to the physician as God phenomenon: "The doctor said, 'Take this,' so I did." That didn't necessarily happen because physicians thought of themselves as gods, although when I interviewed Deepak Chopra, M.D., a few years ago, he commented that some physicians thought the initials M.D. following their names stood for "medical deity."

Women must rise up from this curious supplicant's stance, for how we got there was partly our fault. We women must be ready to admit that it was easier to have someone tell us what to do than to have to gather information ourselves and to think it through. We have enough to think about. But now we must research, think, and act.

The new cohort of women entering the menopausal years wants a physician-partner, not a boss. They want information, not instruction. They want choices, and they want to make their own decisions.

This section of *The Estrogen Answer Book* provides information about the available pharmaceutical estrogen products and answers the questions that women have been asking about the what, when, where, why, and how of estrogen. The first thing to determine, again, is whether or not *you* would benefit from taking estrogen. At this writing, it seems that most women would. However, there are always other points of view, and information derived from various studies, new and old, do not offer bottom-line answers. So before we launch into the different kinds of estrogen products, we need to look again at the latest information on taking estrogen.

62 What recent study shows which women would benefit most from estrogen?

A study reported in the *New England Journal of Medicine* (June 19, 1997) noted that researchers have begun to recognize which women would benefit the most from taking estrogen and who should avoid taking it. The study, conducted by Harvard Medical School and Brigham and Women's Hospital, is based on the Nurses' Study mentioned earlier in this book. That study followed more than 120,000 women who completed questionnaires about their health every other year since 1976. In this research effort, the investigators examined the use of hormones among 3,637 postmenopausal women (a subset of the 120,000 women mentioned above) who died by the end of the research year 1994. The study's leading researcher, Francine Grodstein, noted that two messages emerged from the findings. Number one: women with one or more risk factors for heart disease, such as a family history of the disease, smoking, obesity, high blood pressure, and high cholesterol, can benefit the most from taking estrogen. Number two: if through diet and exercise these women can eliminate their risk factors, they are better off not taking hormones. Huh? That's pretty complicated.

This Harvard study, the most extensive study yet of the effect of estrogen on postmenopausal women, found that ERT reduced the death rate in older women by some *37 percent*, primarily by cutting the risk of death caused by heart disease. Remember, *heart disease is nine times more likely to kill a woman than breast cancer.* The Harvard study also demonstrated that women increased their risk of breast cancer by beginning to take estrogen in their fifties. Can a conclusion be drawn? The one drawn by an editorial in the same issue of the *New England Journal of Medicine* suggests that waiting to begin ERT until a bit later in life might make some sense. Dr. Grodstein notes that although it appears as if healthier women might be better off avoiding hormones, they represent a small minority of the population in general and a small minority in the study. (In the Nurses' Study, the nurse group might have been in better health than the general population.)

Meir J. Stampfer, a Harvard investigator involved in the latest study, admits that this information "changes the risk-benefit equation," noting that women need to make their estrogen decisions based more on other ERT benefits, such as menopause symptom relief and osteoporosis prevention versus increased risk of breast cancer. "It's still very complicated," Dr. Grodstein admits.

Let's look at that 37 percent again and note something significant: According to the study, once a woman had taken HRT or ERT for a decade, the mortality benefit based on heart disease dropped to 20 percent, because the risk from breast cancer rose. Yet, according to Dr. Grodstein, the caveat here is that even women with breast cancer might benefit from estrogen. This study is not a mandate for every woman to be taking hormones, or that there is a specific time limit (such as the ten years mentioned above) to stay on hormones. It is just another in an ongoing series of important studies that seek to nail down answers to this slippery question.

63   In what different forms can estrogen be taken?

There are a number of ways, each working somewhat differently. For example, all estrogen tablets are oral medication, but they are not all the same. For example, Wyeth-Ayerst's Premarin is made up of synthetic conjugated equine estrogen, and Estrace, made by Bristol-Myers Squibb is betadiol-17. Ortho-Est, a product of Ortho-McNeil Pharmaceutical is an estropipate tablet. More about those differences will be covered later in this chapter. The one thing that all oral medications have in common is that they must pass through the liver and be digested before reaching the bloodstream.

Transdermal medications are quite different. They reach the bloodstream through the skin, initially bypassing the liver and thus not changing much on their first pass through the body. That's true as well for some estrogen gels and creams. Injections of course go directly into the bloodstream. There used to be an estrogen pellet that was implanted under the skin, but it was not widely accepted and was taken off the market. There is some thought that it may be reintroduced.

64 I always like to do things in a natural way. What is natural estrogen?

Natural estrogen is probably a misnomer. When it comes to estrogen, "natural" may refer to the hormone made by your own body or it may mean estrogen produced from natural products, and that could include everything from Premarin, which is made from pregnant mare's urine, to one of the patches, such as Climara, which has a soy base, to a full range of phytoestrogens (plant estrogens), which will be covered in chapter 9. Or they may be made from other natural products, like the Mexican yam, by one of the many compounding pharmacies according to your physician's prescription. These pharmacies prepare Bi-Estrogen, which is a combination of about 80 percent estriol (a weaker estrogen) and 20 percent estradiol. They also compound Tri-Estrogen, which is a combination of all three kinds of estrogen that we have had circulating in our bodies: estriol, estradiol, and estrone. Tri-Estrogen can be made up according to your doctor's prescription and adjusted according to your response to it, but it often starts out with 80 percent estriol, 10 percent estradiol, and 10 percent estrone. You can call the National Association of Compounding Pharmacists (see appendix D) to find a compounding pharmacy in your area. If there is none in your area, a call to them, no matter where a pharmacy is located, will bring you and your physician information about those so-called natural compounded products.

65 I have been on Premarin for about ten years. Can you tell me more about the product?

Throughout this book you have seen me refer, as do most people writing about it, to Premarin as the gold standard of estrogen. That is because it has been around for more than fifty-five years. Premarin has not only stood the test of time but has also undergone the greatest amount of testing and research studies, both basic and clinical, of any estrogen product. Premarin has been used in more than three thousand scientific studies concerning estrogen. In fact, it has been the subject of almost 90 percent of the estrogen studies cited in medical literature during the past five years. Of course, Wyeth-Ayerst, the company that makes Premarin, supported many of those studies, but they adhered to scientific principles and practices.

Premarin is an oral tablet and is the number one drug on the market and in patient use. It is the most widely prescribed drug in the United States. Last year more than 45 million prescriptions were written for Premarin. Premarin contains conjugated equine estrogens and got its name from its derivation from pregnant mare's urine.

Not too long ago a member of an audience I was addressing raised her hand and asked me in defiant tones whether I knew what Premarin was made from. When I replied calmly and rather casually that I knew exactly, and said, "The urine from pregnant mares," she dropped the subject. It's one that deserves to be dropped. I have actually visited a couple of the ranches in Canada where pregnant mare's urine is collected and found the care of the horses to be humane and their environment clean and well-kept.

Premarin consists of three major ingredients: estrone sulfate, equilin sulfate, and 17-alpha dihydroequilin sulfate. The estrone sulfate makes up more than half of the product and is a hormone found in both humans and horses. The other products are other estrogens. Premarin is a complex blend of estrogens and is available in five dosage strengths. Interestingly, when a couple of other conjugated estrogens came before the FDA in 1997 they were not proven to be as efficacious as Premarin and did not gain approval, leading researchers to believe that it might well be one of the other estrogens from horses that gives Premarin its unique qualities.

Premarin now comes in several different therapeutic preparations. In addition to the tablet, there is a Premarin vaginal cream, which is helpful for reducing the uncomfortable symptoms of atrophic vaginitis, including burning, itching, and painful intercourse caused by thinning and drying of vaginal tissue resulting from estrogen loss after menopause. The cream helps to restore vaginal tissues' resilience and vaginal pH to normal levels, making women more comfortable and also reducing the risk of vaginal infections.

In 1995 Premarin became available in two new ways for women with an intact uterus who need to take both estrogen and progestin. The new products are Prempro and Premphase. Prempro is the first continuous combined hormone therapy that is two pills in one: estrogen and progestin (medroxyprogesterone acetate) combined, to be taken every single day, 365 days a year. Last year there were more than seven million prescriptions written for Prempro. Premphase is cyclic combined hormone replacement therapy. It works a little differently. The first two weeks of the cycle, the tablet taken contains estrogen alone, the second two weeks, the tablet contains both estrogen and progesterone. Prempro and Premphase are indicated for women who still have their uterus intact.

66 I understand that patches of estrogen bypass my liver, but won't they irritate my skin?

According to an article in the *British Medical Journal* (August 2, 1997), the use of transdermal patches to deliver estrogen may be somewhat limited because of irritation to the skin. The investigators in that study used the two existing forms of estrogen patches. In one, the estrogen is contained in an alcohol reservoir surrounded by an adhesive ring. The example is Estraderm, a patch produced by Novartis Pharmaceuticals. In the other, the estrogen is literally dissolved in the adhesive across the whole patch (called "matrix" patches), examples being Vivelle by Novartis, Alora by Procter & Gamble, and Climara by Berlex Laboratories. It is interesting to note that the study compared the two designs, the reservoir and the matrix, using eighty-two women who had discontinued ERT by patch because of skin irritation.

In the study, women were randomly assigned the reservoir or the matrix patch for eight weeks, and then the other form for another eight weeks (unless skin irritation intervened earlier). Seventy-two participants completed the study. Thirty-three of the women did not stop using either patch; twenty-six discontinued using the reservoir patch; four stopped using the matrix patch; and nine gave up on both patches. The comment at the conclusion was that women who had in the past experienced skin irritation had only a 20 percent chance of experiencing it again with the matrix patch but about a 50 percent chance of renewed skin irritation with the alcohol reservoir patch. Although this was a small study, the authors concluded that for women who had previously given up on the alcohol patch because of skin irritation, the matrix patch might be worth trying.

67 Which kind of patch is Estraderm?

Estraderm was the very first transdermal estrogen product on the market. The development of Estraderm, a product of Ciba Geigy Pharmaceuticals (now Novartis), marked the first real alternative to oral ERT. Estraderm is a twice-weekly transdermal estrogen delivery system that became available in the mid-1980s. That was when women first became aware of through-the-skin, or transdermal, ERT. It heralded the era of no more pills if you had no uterus (women with an intact uterus still required their progestin in tablet form). Estraderm consists of a bubblelike reservoir filled with 17-beta estradiol, which is formulated in an alcohol solution and is designed to deliver estrogen for three to four days. The "bubble" is encircled in adhesive that sticks it to your skin. You change the patch twice each week.

The patch is approximately the size of a silver dollar and is transparent. It is usually worn on various locations on the abdomen or buttocks and delivers estrogen in a slow and steady, even dose. A slightly larger, oval-shaped Estraderm patch contains a larger dose of estrogen. Dosage will be covered in chapter 6.

Enthusiasm for the patch was great. Here was, for the first time, an estrogen delivery system that initially bypassed the liver. That was a good thing, because estrogen taken in tablet form passes through the digestive system, and the liver extensively metabolizes it and may change it in important ways. The theory was and is that bypassing the liver initially made ERT possible for women who had other medical conditions that would preclude their taking it. This meant that women with liver or gallbladder disease, or certain forms of hypertension or other circulatory problems, might consider taking estrogen. Another good feature was that since the estrogen was not initially changed, the physician could more easily monitor it with a simple blood test.

But there were some problems. Women complained about their sensitivity to the adhesive. There was also a complaint, although infrequent, of their skin's sensitivity to the estrogen itself. For most women, these problems could be solved by moving the patch to a new location on the skin each time it is changed. Many women told of a slight or bright pink mark that remained on their skin for days after the patch was changed. For most of these women, with repeated usage the pink mark indicating skin sensitivity simply stopped occurring. Women whose skin continued to be sensitive to the adhesive could switch to another form of estrogen replacement.

There was no doubt, however, that patch therapy was here to stay. A common comment from women was and is "I'm not a great pill taker. I like the way the patch keeps doing its work without me having to remember to take yet another pill." In mid-1998 a new patch, CombiPatch, that contains both estrogen and progestin, became available, eliminating the need for either kind of oral tablet.

68 Does a once-a-week patch like Climara give me enough estrogen?

It does if it works for you. I love the Climara advertisements that say "Forget about menopause for a week." Would that we could! For some women the once-a-week transdermal patch is the answer to their dreams. For other women, the dose is not high enough or does not last through the week, and symptoms reappear when they are least expected, which can be a major bummer. Like other patches, Climara is worn between the waist and the knees and, of course, never on the breasts. The company suggests applying it to the abdomen on clean dry skin and alternating the site of application each week.

Women's bodies respond quite differently to ERT. Individual women are more comfortable with one form of estrogen than another. Climara, as the ad indicates, offers freedom from thinking about medication more than once a week. Climara contains 17-beta estradiol, similar in type to the estrogen naturally produced by the ovaries. Like other transdermal therapy, the estrogen literally goes through the skin into your bloodstream, bypassing the intestinal tract. According to Berlex Laboratories, the company that produces Climara, it is the first, and until recently the only, once-a-week patch. About the size of a half-dollar, extremely thin, and transparent, it is an advanced matrix design, which permits a continuous, even flow of estrogen into the bloodstream.

Climara contains no alcohol, and we're told it has a very low level of skin irritation and lift-off. (According to the company, only 6.8 percent of patients report skin irritation, and fewer than 1 percent note the patch coming off by itself.)

69 What type of estrogen is Alora?

Alora is another patch product, from Procter & Gamble Pharmaceuticals. It, like the other patches, is indicated in the treatment of moderate to severe menopause symptoms. Alora delivers 17-beta estradiol through the skin over a three to four day period through the matrix adhesive formulation. It does not use alcohol. Alora is available in three dose strengths, which offers greater choice in transdermal therapy.

Like other patch products, Alora was tested comparing it with a placebo, with Premarin, and with Climara, and the results were favorable. One study, conducted by TheraTech, Inc., of Salt Lake City, Utah, and Health Decisions, Inc., of Chapel Hill, North Carolina, designed to test Alora against a placebo in post-menopausal women experiencing menopausal symptoms, clearly demonstrated that Alora did its job well. The study showed that the system was effective and safe in the treatment of hot flashes and other symptoms because it delivered estradiol in a range consistent with premenopausal levels, with a low level of skin irritation. So another new choice of ERT became available.

70 Isn't there another new patch called Vivelle, put out by the same company as Estraderm?

You are right, there is. Vivelle became available in the mid-'90s. It is a small transparent patch that you apply directly, on the buttocks or the abdomen, on clean dry skin just like the other patches. It differs from Estraderm in that it is a matrix patch, with the estrogen as part of the edge-to-edge adhesive, rather than the reservoir patch wherein the estrogen is suspended in an alcohol reservoir and an adhesive ring surrounds it. Both patches work well for some women. Here again, as with all other estrogen products, women with an intact uterus require some form of progestin as well; women without a uterus may use estrogen alone.

The same company that makes Vivelle, Novartis Pharma Canada, Inc., has another interesting new product, called Estracomb TTS. Though not available at this time in the United States, Estracomb is a transdermal system (patch) that offers combined replacement of estrogen and progestin. It, like CombiPatch, offers total freedom from tablet taking. Each twenty-eight-day cycle of treatment contains four patches of estradiol for use in weeks 1 and 2 and another four patches that combine estradiol and norethindrone (a type of progestin) acetate to be used in weeks 3 and 4.

71 Is there anything different about a newer product called Fempatch?

This newest of all patches contains a lower dose of estrogen. Fempatch is manufactured by Parke-Davis in a low 0.025 milligram dose thin patch that you change just once a week. It contains 17-beta estradiol, and studies have demonstrated that its low dose is just right for some women, providing them relief from moderate-to-severe menopausal vasomotor symptoms such as hot flashes and night sweats.

72 I hear that just a wee bit of testosterone will rev up my libido. Is that a new idea?

Far from it. Actually, it was noticed back in 1941 when physicians at the University of Chicago won a Nobel Prize for work using testosterone with women with breast cancer. It was noted at that time, although that was not the object of their clinical research, that women on testosterone therapy experience an increase in libido. However, in the 1970s, following the uterine cancer scare connected with the use of estrogen alone, when physicians shunned estrogen, most discarded what they had learned about the relationship of testosterone to increasing libido in women, as well.

But Solvay Pharmaceuticals has been producing Estratest — a tablet combining estrogen and testosterone — for postmenopausal women for years. It's been in use since around 1967, and it was actually "grandfathered" by the FDA. A number of good studies have indicated that both naturally and surgically menopausal women appear to benefit from estrogen-androgen (testosterone) therapy. Because surgical menopause (caused by the removal of the uterus and both ovaries) more sharply decreases both estrogen and androgen hormones than does natural menopause (which is a much slower process), not only might libido vanish, but bone loss might be greatly accelerated as well.

According to Morris Notelovitz, M.D., director of the Women's Medical and Diagnostic Center in Gainesville, Florida, "Their [surgically postmenopausal women's] estrogen levels drop off suddenly, so that they may risk higher than average bone loss than do naturally postmenopausal women." The first long-term, double-blind clinical study comparing the effects of oral estrogen-testosterone therapy with conjugated estrogens (estrogens that have been combined, such as Premarin) in surgically postmenopausal women indicated that treatment with the combination protects against bone loss and relieves menopause symptoms at least as well as the other form of estrogen alone. This clinical trial, conducted by M. Chrystie Timmons, M.D., director of Gerigyn, of Chapel Hill, North Carolina, and colleagues, was reported at a meeting of the North American Menopause Society in November 1996.

Other studies reported at that time showed that women who don't do well on other forms of higher doses of estrogen might benefit from the combination of estrogen and androgen. This may be something women should check out. Another fact to consider is that in the past it was believed that adding the testosterone might lower the cardioprotective effect of the estrogen. It was thought that, since research has shown that estrogen raised high density lipoprotein (HDL, the "good" cholesterol), which may be one of the reasons that estrogen protects women's hearts, and since testosterone is known to lower HDL, the combination pill might just offset the heart-healthy effects of the estrogen. Another study reported at that same NAMS meeting said that "Androgens aren't bad — they just may have a neutral effect on atherosclerosis." See what your own physician thinks.

In the meantime, many of the women I've talked with said that within a week of starting Estratest their libido came roaring back. Other women noted no change at all. If lack of libido is your problem and heart disease is not, you might want to try Estratest and see how it affects you. There are also other ways to take testosterone, such as by injection, pellet placed under the skin of the buttock, or compounded tablet or capsule.

73   What's Estratab?

That's another estrogen tablet made by Solvay Pharmaceutical, only without the testosterone. It is a plant-based estrogen that comes in three dose sizes. See the chart in chapter 6. A recent study of this product demonstrated that a very low dose of estrogen (0.3 milligram per day) not only increased bone mineral density but also alleviated menopause symptoms without increasing the risk of endometrial hyperplasia (overgrowth of the lining of the uterus.) This low dose is about half the amount of estrogen formerly thought to offer protection against osteoporosis, according to Dr. Notelovitz. He noted that although he might have suspected that the lowest possible dose of estrogen would cause the fewest cases of endometrial hyperplasia, he was surprised to find that the low dose also offered protection against osteoporosis.

74   What is the new estrogen ring I've been hearing about?

If your major menopause problem is urogenital atrophy, this new prescription product called Estring, available since January 1997 from Pharmacia & Upjohn Pharmaceuticals, may be right for you. Urogenital atrophy is a fancy medical way of saying that you are experiencing vaginal thinning and drying from lack of lubrication, and pain with sexual intercourse as a result. It may also mean that you are experiencing other urinary problems having to do with frequency — the sense you must urinate all the time or, at least, too often — urgency — the sense that you won't make it to the powder room in time — and stress incontinence — the problem with leaking a little urine when you cough, sneeze, laugh too heartily, or work out too strenuously.

Estring is a soft, flexible ring, containing low-dose estrogen, that is inserted into the vagina like a contraceptive diaphragm. It places estrogen in the vagina, like vaginal creams, but it has some major advantages. Because of its unique continous-release system, an Estring once in place lasts ninety days and is not messy, and most women and men say they cannot feel the ring during intercourse. Estring is as effective as the vaginal creams, which can be messy and which often need to be applied once a day (tapering off to one to three times a week for some women). With Estring you can insert it and forget it for a while. The level of estrogen in Estring is extremely low, and inasmuch as it acts only on the tissues of the lower vaginal and urinary tract, women with an intact uterus need not take any form of progestin or progesterone with it. When you first use Estring it may take up to three weeks for you to experience significant improvement.

75 Can't over-the-counter vaginal lubricants do the same job of returning lubrication as Estring?

Yes they can, and they do it well for women who have only slight problems with lubrication. They are important to know about, since using petroleum jelly, baby oil, or other oils or cosmetic creams and lotions can upset the vagina's delicately balanced environment and should not be used. Good choices of nonhormonal over-the-counter vaginal lubricants and moisturizers include the following:

Astroglide, by Biofilm Laboratories
Gyne-Moistrin, by Shering-Plough Health Care Products
Replens, by Warner-Lambert
Lubrin, by Kenwood Laboratories
Moist Again, by Lake Pharmaceuticals
K-Y Jelly, by Johnson and Johnson

76 What exactly are SERMs?

SERM is an acronym for a brand new class of drugs called Selective Estrogen Receptor Modulators. They are an innovative and exciting new entry into the arena of women's health preservation.

Eli Lilly and Company, in its Indianapolis-based Pharmaceutical Division, presented data on its SERM in Washington, D.C., at the Fourth International Symposium on Osteoporosis Research Advances and Clinical Applications sponsored by the National Osteoporosis Foundation in June 1997. Lilly's new compound, raloxifene, was studied for the prevention of osteoporosis and offers a new choice to women. The compound can act like estrogen in the bones and cardiovascular system and at the same time block estrogenic effects in the breasts and uterus.

Raloxifene was studied in more than twelve thousand women in more than twenty-five countries. The results were excellent. Raloxifene, compared with a placebo, over a period of twenty-four months, prevented bone loss in the spine and hip, significantly increasing bone mineral density. According to Ethel Siris, M.D., director of the Osteoporosis Center at Columbia University, "Preserving this bone mass is critical to maintaining a woman's long-term health and vitality after menopause, by decreasing her risk of disabling fractures as she ages."

The effects of raloxifene on lipids and other indicators for heart attacks and strokes were also evaluated throughout the clinical trials. Studies demonstrated that raloxifene reduced LDL (low-density lipoprotein, the "bad" cholesterol) but did not alter HDL or triglycerides. It also reduced fibrinogen (a coagulation factor in the blood), which when elevated has been suggested as an additional risk factor for heart disease. More research into raloxifene's long-term effect on the heart is under way.

In the uterus, raloxifene did not stimulate tissue growth, nor did it cause spotting or bleeding. Raloxifene also did not stimulate breast tissue in women, and did not cause breast swelling, tenderness, or pain. Both stimulation of the uterine lining, causing potentially precancerous growth, and breast stimulation may occur in some women on HRT or ERT.

Hot flashes did not fare as well in the studies. Women taking raloxifene reported a slightly higher rate of hot flashes than women taking a placebo, yet hot flashes caused very few women (2 percent) to discontinue raloxifene.

Raloxifene received FDA approval on December 9, 1997. By January 1998 it was available at pharmacies under the name Evista. It represents a significant addition to the armamentarium women have in protecting their long-term health. This newest drug will offer women who cannot take estrogen for medical reasons, or who choose not to take it for whatever reasons, a new approach to protecting their bones and their hearts as well as their uterus and breasts, all at the same time.

It is very exciting that so many new forms of HRT and ERT and now SERMs have become available for postmenopausal women. These may truly enable us to live better while we're living longer. It is important that each woman keep herself fully informed of all of her options so that she can make the best decisions for herself. You might need to bring the latest information to your physician, since, as I've mentioned, many of them initially prescribe the same medication in the same dose for about 90 percent of their patients. You don't want to be included in that 90 percent; you want your prescribed product custom-tailored to your specific needs. So it is important for you to insist on individualized care. There are more products, in more strengths, than ever before when it comes to replacing diminished or lost hormones. If one product doesn't work well for you, consider another. If one dosage doesn't do the trick, ask your physician to help you fiddle with dosage until it works just right. Don't settle for less.

6

What Are the Dosages
of Estrogen?

W HEN I travel and lecture and interview women, a familiar refrain haunts our conversations: "The pill [or the
patch] I was on wasn't helping me. I still had hot flashes
and I wasn't sleeping well either. Then I read another
article about breast cancer in the newspaper, so I quit taking estrogen. No, I didn't call my physician first. What for? There's
nothing else for me to take, right?" Wrong. As you read in chapter 5, there is a vast array of products that can ease or eliminate
menopause symptoms and that offer protection from long-term
health problems. Ask your physician about them. Typically if estrogen is working for you, your symptoms should diminish in one
week and disappear in two weeks. As you will learn when you
read on, some preparations are available in one or two strengths;
others come in three, four, or five strengths, leaving even more
room for experimenting with what dose will really work for you.

For example, Premarin comes in five strengths — 0.3, .625,
.90, 1.25, and 2.5 milligrams. Estraderm, the patch, comes in two
doses, .05 and .10. There is no magic formula for which dose
your physician prescribes for you, except what works. So, most
doctors who prescribe Premarin will start out with .625, because
the smaller dose was not shown until recently to be enough to
prevent osteoporosis.

Now, .625 will work for some women, but not for others. So women call their physicians and the dosage is adjusted up or down until the right strength is found or until the women give up and say "Forget about estrogen." Most women don't say those words directly to their doctors. What they do most often is accept the new prescription for the higher or lower strength and never fill it.

A patient satisfaction survey was done by Stephen A. Brunton, M.D., clinical professor of family medicine, University of California at Irvine, and reported in *Today's Therapeutic Trends 1996*, which showed why there is often a lack of compliance. The study was called "Estrogen Replacement Therapy (ERT): Results of a Patient Satisfaction Survey of Women Receiving ERT and Implications for Treatment." Its objective was to confirm findings from previous clinical studies showing that not all women experience complete symptom relief as a result of ERT and to assess women's satisfaction with their current forms of ERT (with a view toward discussing treatment options).

The results were not surprising. The two hundred women currently using oral forms of ERT who responded to the telephone survey said that their most pressing reason for starting ERT was to eliminate hot flashes and night sweats. Sixty-four percent of the women were using Premarin and 21 percent were taking Estrace. Three-fourths of the women surveyed were between the ages of forty-one and sixty; 11 percent were age forty or younger, and 15 percent were older than sixty. More than one-third of the women surveyed reported that they had their estrogen prescription changed at least once, and more than two-thirds of them had changed because their form of ERT was not providing relief from symptoms.

Let's review the results. When women were asked why they had started ERT they said they wanted relief from or were concerned about:

hot flashes and night sweats	73 percent
osteoporosis prevention/treatment	55 percent
mood swings	54 percent
vaginal dryness	42 percent

fatigue	40 percent
insomnia	39 percent
menstrual changes	27 percent

What is most troubling is that 47 percent of the women said that they did not discuss with their physicians their persistent menopause symptoms while on ERT. I urge women to get right back to their physicians if they are not getting symptom relief with their prescription. It is not complaining when you say to your doctor "This isn't working for me. Let's try something else." That's a lot better than simply stopping your therapy without notifying your doctor. In fact, if you want or need to stop, don't do it cold turkey. The answer to question 21 in chapter 2 gives some suggestions about how to slowly come off ERT or HRT. Review those options with your physician, who may have an even better plan.

See the charts at the end of this chapter for strengths in which each ERT and HRT product is available. You should understand the strength of each product and the pros and cons of various doses. Here, again, an informed woman is far more likely to seek help when she knows there *is* help.

77 **How many different strengths does Premarin come in, and what are the pluses and minuses of each?**

As mentioned earlier, Premarin, the oral tablet, comes in five different dosage strengths. Premarin at this writing is the most widely prescribed drug in the United States and has been for many years. It also has an impressive presence throughout the world. There was some concern that its smallest dose, 0.3 milligram, which is a dark green oval tablet, might not have significant bone protecting effect. It has not been studied for cardioprotective effect, though it can result in symptom relief for some women. The most commonly prescribed dose is .625 milligram, a dark-red oval tablet. From that dose the prescription can be raised or lowered according to the patient's requirements. Premarin should make hot flashes and night sweats lessen or disappear and should increase vaginal lubrication, reducing the risk of vaginal infections and making intercourse comfortable again. The other three doses are higher. There

is a white tablet containing 0.9 milligram, a yellow tablet containing 1.25 milligrams, and a purple tablet of 2.5 milligrams. There
may be a Premarin dose to make every woman comfortable.

78 **I take Estrace, a tiny lavender pill, but sometimes it doesn't
seem to relieve me of those hot, hot flashes. Should I take
something else?**

Estrace comes in more than one strength. The lavender
pill you are taking is the 1 milligram size. Estrace also comes in
a turquoise pill that is 2 milligrams or double the strength you
are using. Discuss increasing the dose with your physician. Sometimes you only have to increase the dose for a brief period of
time. I have talked to many women who have over ten or fifteen
years on HRT or ERT changed doses many times. It seems that
sometimes our bodies can simply get used to a drug and sometimes it stops working as effectively as it did. I know many
women who over the years make changes as soon as their comfort
level diminishes. I know more women who either keep taking a
preparation with minimal success or who just give up estrogen
altogether. In light of all the research into the long-term benefits
of estrogen that seems like a mistake to me.

79 **I am taking Premarin, 0.625 milligram for twenty-five days,
and adding 10 milligrams of Provera [a progestin] for the last
twelve days. Then I discontinue both drugs and get my period.
I don't mind the period as much as the PMS that begins shortly
after I start the Provera. Can't the doses be adjusted in some
way so that I don't have PMS for the rest of my life?**

The doses can and should be adjusted. Often when we get
the bloating, the emotional nasties, and the crying need to eat
everything that isn't under lock and key, it's time to look carefully
at the progestin we are taking. As mentioned earlier, estrogen is
said to have a mental tonic effect, but progestin can be the hormone of the PMS blues. It is often the villain. Talk to your physician about cutting down on the progestin (many women take
just 5 milligrams) or about changing the form of progestin you are

taking. For example, the oral micronized progesterone prepared by a compounding pharmacy from your physician's prescription usually minimizes PMS or makes it disappear completely. Some physicians believe that there is no magic to taking progestin every month and suggest taking it every other month or quarterly.

Then there are women like my friend Elizabeth. She is so miserable on the progestin that she doesn't take it at all, opting instead for an endometrial sampling in her gynecologist's office every six months to make sure there is no buildup of endometrium. You can also think about a change in regimen altogether. In chapter 7 you'll find information about a continuous regimen of estrogen and progestin (taken in a very low dose) that may do away with the PMS and, over six months or so, end your monthly menstrual periods as well.

Whatever you choose to do, do something. There is no reason to suffer like the many women who are unaware that there are so many choices to consider.

80 What is the simplest way to take HRT?

I have to say that Prempro is probably the simplest. A Prempro tablet contains 0.625 milligram of conjugated equine estrogen and 2.5 milligrams of medroxyprogesterone acetate (a synthetic progestin). You take one each day every day of the year. Some women tell me of problems with breakthrough spotting or bleeding, but most women tell me they love the simplicity of one pill.

Prempro is the product used in the HERS trial (see question 56). According to Stephen B. Hulley, M.D., professor at UCSF and leader of the study, "Based on these findings, we don't recommend starting HRT for the purpose of preventing heart attacks in postmenopausal women with existing heart disease. There was no overall benefit during the four years of the trial, and the risk of heart attacks seemed to increase soon after starting hormones. But women who are already taking HRT could continue, given the apparent decrease in risk of heart attack after several years." Other physicians suggest the study may have been too short to demonstrate benefits. Stay tuned.

81 **I'm looking for a very low dose estrogen, just enough to stop these darn hot flashes and night sweats. At this point I don't care about long-term symptoms, I just want to get over this hot, sweaty stuff. Can anything help me?**

In 1997 a new low-dose estrogen patch called Fempatch became available. It delivers a very low dose of estradiol, just 0.025 milligram. Best of all, you use one patch for an entire week. This may be just the right dose for getting rid of your hot flashes and night sweats. Fempatch is also reported to help with vaginal dryness. The only drawback to Fempatch is that this low dose of estrogen may not provide protection from osteoporosis or heart disease.

82 **I've been on the Estraderm patch for about five years and have had some problems with the doses. Sometimes the 0.05 is not enough to counteract my symptoms, and yet I haven't been willing to double up and go on the only other size it comes in, 0.1 milligram. So I have sometimes used the larger patch and put tape over part of it to get a dose somewhere between the two. Now the company has come out with another patch that has a midpoint, or three-quarter dose. I'm confused about what to do. Can you clear up my confusion?**

Estraderm was the first transdermal system of estrogen replacement approved by the FDA in the mid-1980s — the first patch. It still comes in two dosages, 0.05 and 0.1 milligram. It is a reservoir patch, as described in chapter 5. In 1996 the same company developed another estradiol patch and called it Vivelle. It is a matrix patch, meaning the estrogen and adhesive are mixed together. Vivelle is somewhat smaller than Estraderm and comes in four dosages, or strengths: 0.375, 0.05, 0.075, and 0.1 milligram, allowing for more dosing flexibility. That may be your answer to the in-between-size dose. Some women swear by Estraderm; others like Vivelle and find that it causes no skin irritation and permits their dose to be better tailored to their needs. Both Vivelle and Estraderm are changed twice each week.

83 I cannot stand messing with estrogen vaginal cream every couple of days, but if I don't, I've got real problems. I need to run to the bathroom every two minutes with the fear I won't get there in time, and the prospect of painful intercourse makes me want to stay in the bathroom all night. I've tried estrogen suppositories; they're too messy too. Isn't there a low dose of something that I can use?

Estring, a new-to-the-market flexible estrogen ring, can be inserted into the vagina and left there for ninety days. It will deliver a continuous dose of estrogen and should relieve vaginal dryness and urinary urgency. Estring delivers such a low dose of estrogen, 2 milligrams total over the ninety days, that, according to Mary K. Beard, M.D., associate clinical professor of obstetrics/gynecology at the University of Utah, it has little effect on breast or uterine tissue and may be an option for women who have a personal or a family history of breast cancer.

84 Help, please. I'm taking estrogen but am still experiencing menopause symptoms and I'm miserable. I've heard that hot flashes, night sweats, and a dry, itchy vagina are called the nuisance symptoms of menopause. They are more than a nuisance to me — they are absolutely diminishing the good quality of my life. What can I do?

You've got to go back to your physician's office and complain that your brand and dose of estrogen is not alleviating your symptoms. Take a look at the end of this chapter and you will see a table of estrogen products including pills, patches, creams, and even a vaginal ring. Note how many different doses these products come in — undoubtedly there's one right for you.

It remains very interesting to me that bright, active women are not fully aware of the facts about estrogen, and that includes knowing there are different products, manufactured from different estrogen sources, available in different strengths. This is not a woman's fault, this is the fault of the physician who, as we learned earlier, may start all patients on one drug in one strength.

I can almost understand that prescribing formula. It's easier for the physician, and for many women it works. As Dr. R. Jeffrey Chang explains, "Physicians often become comfortable with one product, know everything about it, and because of their knowledge prescribe it most often." The problem is that for other women it doesn't work, and then it becomes the woman's responsibility to get back to the physician and complain loud and clear about persistent symptoms. It helps if you, the patient, have that conversation fully armed with information about what else there is that you can try.

85 Will taking vitamin E along with my estrogen help get rid of persistent hot flashes?

It's important to be familiar with vitamin E in this regard, because although at this writing there is no solid scientific proof that vitamin E counteracts hot flashes and night sweats, it does work that way for many women. I know this is what is frowned upon as anecdotal evidence, but it is important that you are aware of the properties of vitamin E. (Chapters 10 and 11 contain more about vitamin E, and other vitamins and minerals that can help.) Please be aware that taking megadoses of anything can be risky. Vitamin E is often contraindicated for women with high blood pressure, diabetes, or a rheumatic heart condition, and it should not be taken at all by anyone who is taking digitalis.

86 Is there a difference in the amount of estrogen in birth control pills and that used in ERT?

There is a major difference. Even the new low-dose birth control pills contain a great deal more estrogen than the amount used in ERT or HRT to make menopause symptoms diminish or disappear. Estrogen replacement is not usually prescribed for women with a history of inflammation of a vein (phlebitis) or a blood clot (an embolism), particularly if it was related to taking birth control pills.

Birth control pills have also been known to raise blood pressure, which postmenopausal ERT does not appear to do, but your physician will undoubtedly check your blood pressure at every visit. If your blood pressure does seem to elevate, your doctor may ask you to switch from an oral tablet to one of the many estrogen patches, because in initially bypassing the liver, the patch may resolve the elevated blood pressure issue.

87 How do most physicians generally decide what dose of estrogen to start a woman on?

I have discussed this subject with many physicians. Most of them will determine where to begin ERT depending on the severity of your symptoms and your health status and taking into consideration your personal and family medical history. Typically, a doctor will start at a midpoint, see how the dose works for you, and then alter it as necessary. However, you have a responsibility here, too. It is important that you keep your physician informed about how well you are tolerating the dosage and whether or not it has only somewhat reduced or entirely eliminated your menopause symptoms. Getting the estrogen prescription just right is a two-way street. You report, the physician listens, and together you choose the next dose to try.

The chart that follows gives dosages for the most widely used estrogen preparations.

THE MOST WIDELY USED ESTROGEN PREPARATIONS

Brand Name	Active Ingredients	Dosage	Color	Manufacturer
ORAL ESTROGENS				
Estrace	micronized estradiol	1 mg 2 mg	lilac turquoise	Bristol-Myers Squibb (in Canada, Roberts)
Estratab	esterified estrogen	0.3 mg 0.625 mg 1.25 mg 2.5 mg	blue yellow red purple	Solvay
Estrovis	quinestrol	0.1 mg	light blue	Parke-Davis
Menest	esterified estrogen	0.3 0.625 1.25	yellow orange green	SmithKline Beecham
Ogen	estropipate	0.625 mg	yellow	Pharmacia & Upjohn
Ortho-Est	estropipate	0.625 mg 1.25 mg	orange lavender	Ortho-McNeil
Premarin	conjugated equine estrogens	0.3 mg 0.625 mg 0.9 mg 1.25 mg 2.5 mg	dark green dark red white yellow purple	Wyeth-Ayerst
ESTROGEN PATCHES				
Alora	estradiol (matrix)	0.05 mg 0.075 mg 0.1 mg	clear	Procter & Gamble
Climara	estradiol (matrix)	0.5 mg 0.1 mg	clear	Berlex
CombiPatch (new)	estradiol with norethindrone	50/140 mcg 50/250 mcg	clear	Rhône-Poulenc Rorer
Estraderm	estradiol (reservoir)	0.05 mg 0.1 mg	clear	Novartis
Fempatch	estradiol (matrix)	0.025 mg	clear	Parke-Davis
Vivelle	estradiol (matrix)	0.375 mg 0.05 mg 0.075 mg 0.1 mg	clear	Novartis
ESTROGEN RING				
Estring	estradiol	2.0 mg		Pharmacia & Upjohn
ESTROGEN COMPOUND				
Evista	raloxifene	60 mg	white	Eli Lilly

Brand Name	Active Ingredients	Dosage	Color	Manufacturer
ESTROGEN CREAM (FOR VAGINAL USE)				
Estrace	estradiol	0.1 mg in 1 g cream		Bristol-Meyers Squibb
Ogen	estropipate	1.5 mg in 1 g cream		Pharmacia & Upjohn
Ortho	dienestrol	0.01 percent		Ortho-McNeil
Premarin	conjugated equine estrogens	0.625 mg in 1 g cream		Wyeth-Ayerst
ESTROGEN COMBINED WITH TESTOSTERONE				
Estratest	esterified estrogens	1.25 mg	dark green	Solvay
	with methyl-testosterone	2.5 mg		
Estratest H.S.	esterified estrogens	0.625 mg	light green	Solvay
	with methyl-testosterone	1.25 mg		
ESTROGEN COMBINED WITH PROGESTIN				
Prempro	conjugated equine estrogens	0.625 mg	peach	Wyeth-Ayerst
	with medroxy-progesterone acetate	2.5 mg		
Premphase (2 tablets)	conjugated equine estrogens	0.625 mg	maroon	Wyeth-Ayerst
	with medroxy-progesterone acetate	2.5 mg	light blue	
PROGESTINS AND PROGESTERONE				
Amen	medroxy-progesterone acetate	5 mg 10 mg	peach/white peach/white	Reed & Carnrick
Aygestin	norethindrone acetate	5 mg	white	ESI Lederle
Cycrin	medroxy-progesterone acetate	2.5 mg 5 mg 10 mg	white lilac peach	ESI Lederle
Norlutate	norethindrone acetate	5 mg	pink	Parke-Davis
Provera	medroxy-progesterone acetate	2.5 mg 5 mg 10 mg	orange white white (round)	Pharmacia & Upjohn

In addition to the progestins and progesterone listed on page 112, oral micronized progesterone can be compounded by a pharmacist according to your physician's prescription. Because of the small particles these compounds contain, many women are relieved of progestin's side effects. Talk with your physician. Other hormones, such as estrogen and testosterone, can also be compounded by one of the many compounding pharmacies. I will explain this more fully in part III.

There is also a new choice, Crinone by Columbia Laboratories. This is a vaginally delivered progesterone gel, approved by the FDA for use with infertility that is prescribed off label (meaning without FDA approval for this purpose) for use in HRT. Crinone is the first product to deliver progesterone directly to the uterus, maximizing therapeutic benefits. According to James Lie, M.D., professor of obstetrics and gynecology and director of reproductive endocrinology, University of Cincinnati, writing in *Menopause Management* (July/August 1997), "It [Crinone] allows progesterone to be absorbed very efficiently through the vagina. And, yes, this may ultimately be an answer with respect to use in the postmenopausal regimen."

The FDA recently approved a micronized natural progesterone called Prometrium, which is a product of Solvay Pharmaceuticals, for use in secondary amenorrhea, but an application is in review for its use in HRT. Prometrium is identical in structure to women's naturally occurring progesterone and may eliminate a lot of the problems that some women have with Provera (a synthetic progestin). Some physicians are already prescribing it for use in HRT off label. So Prometrium capsules join oral micronized progesterone preparations from compounding pharmacies as the only forms of progesterone available in the United States. Prometrium was originally introduced in France and is widely used in Europe. It is approved for marketing in more than twenty-five countries worldwide.

7

What Different Regimens Can I Consider?

ONCE you decide that estrogen is for you and you've learned about the many products and their strengths, the next thing you need to think about is what regimen (or prescribing plan) you are going to follow. Here again, before you choose it is important that you know of and understand the many different ways you can take estrogen. And when you decide which one to start with, keep in mind that your choice need not be a forever one. It's as easy to change regimens as it is to switch products or doses. Nothing works for everybody. Getting estrogen right for you can take several adjustments and some fine-tuning. Never hesitate to contact your physician and say, "This is not working well for me, let's try something else." Don't be embarrassed, don't think you are bothering the doctor too much; just think about feeling great and perhaps living longer and better once the estrogen puzzle is properly solved for you. Ideally, you are working toward estrogen replacement therapy that is comfortable for you, that eliminates symptoms, and that gives you no negative side effects. You are the only person who can know what works best for you, and it is your job to keep communicating with your doctor until together you get it right.

Until you do, there may be fits and starts and disappointment and discomfort. I'd like to suggest that trying on estrogen is like having a coat or suit or evening gown designed and custom-made especially for you. Frequent fittings and consultations ensue until the garment is perfect for you. Consider that the scenario when you seek ERT. If it doesn't fit or feel right, then, like a gown, it needs to be adjusted in some way. Now that you know how many different ways estrogen can be taken, you can see how many different ways it can be adjusted. I know the adjustments can be bothersome, but when short-term relief and long-term good health are your goals, it is worth it.

88 My uterus is still with me and I know I need HRT, comprised of both estrogen and progestin. What kinds of therapeutic regimens can I consider?

Even though you need to protect the lining of your uterus by taking both female sex hormones, there are still different ways to accomplish that. The most common regimens in your case are sequential combined therapy and continuous combined therapy.

The sequential approach is an attempt to mimic your own premenopausal menstrual cycle. The first day of the month you take estrogen and plan to take it for a total of twenty-five days. Between day 13 and day 15 or 16 — whichever you and your doctor decide on — you add the progestin. You take both the estrogen and progestin until day 25 and then stop both medications. When you stop, you will begin "withdrawal" bleeding. That simply means you have withdrawn the medications and when you do, a menstrual period will occur. (Should bleeding occur at any other time — called "break-through" bleeding — notify your physician immediately.)

Having a period on the sequential therapy makes sense, because you are literally taking the hormones in much the same way your body produced and sequenced them since puberty. A number of women have told me, "I like having my period, it keeps me feeling young." Other women say, "I was counting on being done with the mess and bother of it all and here I am, still running out for Tampax." For these women there are other choices, although the sequential method, tampons and all, is the regimen that's been around the longest.

The newer method that does eventually eliminate menstrual periods is the continuous combined therapy, in which you take both estrogen and progestin every day of the year. No starting, no stopping, and usually no period after about six months or a year. Again, that's the good news. The bad news is that there can be a lot of erratic bleeding during that first six months, and many women don't want to deal with the sheer irregularity of it. I've read that one in two women who start the continuous combined therapy stop it before their menstrual bleeding ceases. Older women starting continuous combined therapy may experience fewer problems with bleeding and so may be more likely to stay with this regimen. The differences in bleeding, according to Isaac Shiff, M.D., chief of obstetrics and gynecology at Massachusetts General Hospital, is probably because the uterine lining in older women is less responsive to the hormones. How best to take HRT is yet another area begging for more research.

Other, less frequently used regimens of HRT work with some success for some women. I am aware of regimens in which the progestin is added to the estrogen for the first twelve days of the month. Menstruation-like bleeding often occurs after day 10. This works for some women, because they appreciate knowing the bleeding schedule. In another regimen, estrogen is used continuously and progestins are added for three days, stopped for three days, and added again for three days, and this pattern is repeated all month. When I described the possibility of this regimen working for them, some women said to me, "That would make me crazy! I'd never know what I was doing!" That may be true, yet of the tiny number of women studied who were on this pattern, none experienced bleeding after the first twelve months of therapy.

The regimen that seems to me the most comfortable is one in which estrogen is used continuously every day of every month and progestin is added only every third month for ten to thirteen or fourteen days. Your period may be heavier, but it occurs only quarterly, and with appropriate checking by your physician this might prove to be enough to protect the lining of the uterus from excessive tissue buildup. I remember hearing Malcolm Pike, M.D., say at a meeting of the North American Menopause Society a few years ago that there is no magic in giving progestin every month and that other suitable and safe regimens were possible. Talk to your own physician and see what can be worked out for you.

89 My uterus is intact, but I cannot bear the progestins. They make me blue and miserable. Can't I forego progestin and just take estrogen?

Maybe yes, maybe no. You might be able to if your doctor agrees and you are on a very low dose of estrogen and agree to have regular endometrial samplings. (There is vast disagreement among the women I have discussed the samplings with; some say they experience no pain, others say they found them quite painful.) I do believe, if the side effects of the progestin are unbearable for you, that carefully watched estrogen alone with regular examination of your endometrium may be a solution. Check it out. Also check out the oral micronized progesterone available from compounding pharmacies with your physician's prescription, and Crinone, a natural progesterone in vaginal gel form that some physicians use in HRT off label (see page 113). (Off label means Crinone was not approved by the FDA for that purpose, even though it was approved as a treatment for infertility and for the absence of periods in women who had menstruated regularly.)

90 With no uterus to worry about, can I just take any type of estrogen?

You can, and you can take it in a couple of ways. You can take it for twenty-five days a month and take a week off, or you can take it continuously and not have to think about a schedule at all. If you choose to stop for a week, you may find your symptoms racing back, so many women don't think it's worth stopping at all. I know when I've stopped estrogen, by day 3. I suffer hot flashes and the mother of all night sweats, and by mid-week my heart palpitations come pounding back. It may be worth a try, however, just to see whether or not you've become free of symptoms. I have not.

91   What's the hormone "cocktail" I've been hearing about?

Why the addition of testosterone, the so-called male hormone turned hormone therapy into a cocktail I'll never know. I do know, though, that testosterone is the hormone of desire and if added to your hormone replacement therapy, it should be taken in conjunction with estrogen.

According to Estelle Ramey, M.D., professor emeritus, Georgetown University School of Medicine, all women do not experience a loss of libido after menopause, but some 30 percent do. For those women, and I have interviewed many of them, the lack of sexual desire is devastating. One woman said to me recently, "I just lie there beside my partner of more than thirty-five years and feel nothing. Oh, sure, I love him and care for him. I just feel no physical desire. I'm grateful when I fall asleep or he does without having to deal with trying to be intimate. I didn't think this was what getting older was all about."

Well, there is something that can be done. Just a little bit of testosterone can bring back your former sexy self. I know it is difficult to talk to your doctor about this really important issue, but talk you must if you want help. I believe that our physicians should always ask two questions about our sex lives during our examination or consultation: Are you sexually active? and Are you sexually satisfied? Most often they don't, so you have to bite the bullet and bring up the subject of your lost libido. If you're uncomfortable talking about it, write out your questions and hand them to your doctor. Anything that gets the conversation going is a good idea.

In the answer to question 31 in chapter 3, I described how testosterone can work for you and why women may lose the little bit we have when we lose our other hormones at menopause.

Maybe you should consider adding testosterone to your ERT or HRT. When it is prescribed, testosterone is often given in the same regimen as your estrogen, except in the case of the testosterone by injection or pellet. The injection lasts about one month, the pellet, usually inserted under the skin of the buttock, lasts approximately three months. But there are estrogen-testosterone combination pills as well. Estratest has been around since the 1960s and has certainly stood the test of time. This tablet type of estrogen-androgen combination (both estrogen and testosterone) includes esterified estrogens and methyltestosterone. The injection usually contains estradiol cypionate and testosterone cypionate. According to a reproductive endocrinologist in southern California, Ted Quigley, who was an early proponent of testosterone replacement for women, the testosterone pellet is actually composed of a soy product. What could be more natural?

8

What's New in Hormone Replacement Therapy?

JUST when we think we know what's out there to help women through menopause and the many years beyond, a new compound appears. The one called raloxifene, mentioned earlier, is very exciting. It is the first of what are glibly being called "designer estrogens" in the media hype. The word "designer," however, doesn't refer to Donna Karan or Calvin Klein. It does refer to a new class of drugs called selective estrogen receptor modulators, or SERMs.

To add to the confusion, SERMs are not hormones but can act like hormones in certain select places in the body, for example our bones and hearts, and *not* act like estrogen in our breasts and uterus. The idea of designer estrogens is fairly apt, referring as it does to the ability of this compound to select how and when to act like estrogen and when to inhibit estrogen's effect.

SERMs have the ability to act on different estrogen receptor cells in completely different ways. Estrogen receptors, you will recall, can be likened to locks on cells. SERMs can be the key to unlocking estrogen receptor cells in some areas, like the skeleton and the cardiovascular system, and yet be unable to unlock and get themselves into other estrogen receptors on cells elsewhere in the body. For example, they can't say "open sesame" and get into the uterus and the breasts.

What does this mean? It may mean that women who are fearful of replacing estrogen because they are worried about breast cancer might be interested in trying this type of compound. When we consider that fewer than 20 percent of menopausal and postmenopausal women use HRT or ERT, we must realize that either they cannot take it for medical reasons or choose not to take it because of fear of one kind or another. Consider SERMs another battle won in the ongoing struggle to provide replacement medications to protect women as they age.

Raloxifene, this newest SERM, was launched early in January 1998 after receiving approval from the FDA on December 9, 1997. But it is not really the first SERM. In fact, around the middle of the 1980s we began to hear about another SERM, called tamoxifen. Although it was not classified as a SERM or designer anything back then, tamoxifen, used primarily for breast cancer patients because it has anti-estrogenic effects on breast tissue and is able to compete with estrogen at receptor sites (the lock-and-key approach), where it becomes bound to the site and inhibits cancerous cells from spreading and taking over other cells. So the use of tamoxifen, with its estrogen-blocking ability in the breast has been important in controlling breast cancer. Conversely, tamoxifen also has the ability to act like estrogen in the skeleton and on the cardiovascular system, protecting bones, though not quite as well as estrogen, and hearts, by maintaining good cholesterol levels. Tamoxifen has its negative side, too. It has been demonstrated to cause endometrial cancer because of its estrogenic effects in the uterus. Some women taking tamoxifen after breast cancer found that it exacerbated hot flashes. Further, studies began to show that while short term (about five years) use of tamoxifen was breast protective, taking it for ten years was bordering on dangerous, because that was when it began to stimulate the tissues of the breast. Tamoxifen, then, it must be noted, has both estrogenic and anti-estrogenic effects.

Then along came two important developments concerning tamoxifen that excited the scientific community and women worldwide. First, on April 30, 1998, Zeneca Pharmaceuticals announced that it had submitted a supplemental new drug application to the Food and Drug Administration for the use of its tamoxifen citrate product (Nolvadex) in the prevention of breast cancer in women at increased risk for the disease. The submission followed a decision by the National Cancer Institute and the National Surgical Adjuvant Breast and Bowel Project to call an early halt to the Breast Cancer Prevention Trial, which was to have been a five-year study of Nolvadex versus a placebo in women at increased risk of developing breast cancer. The trial was stopped because of favorable finding for the prevention of breast cancer.

That announcement was followed by one on May 14, 1998, reporting on a fifteen-year international analysis that showed that Nolvadex has the potential for saving the lives of thousands of breast cancer patients. This study, which included fifty-five randomized trials with thirty-seven thousand women, demonstrated that five years of tamoxifen therapy substantially reduced the recurrence of breast cancer and improved the ten-year survival rate for all patients regardless of age, menopausal status, or whether or not they had received chemotherapy treatment.

Back in June 1997 the FDA had approved another product for the treatment of metastatic breast cancer. Fareston, by Shering Plough, is a once-a-day oral anti-estrogen that binds to estrogen receptors in cancer cells and blocks estrogen from further stimulating tumor growth. Fareston is indicated for postmenopausal women with estrogen-receptor-positive or unknown tumors. The chemical structure of Fareston is different from that of tamoxifen, but both drugs are anti-estrogens.

How have SERMs changed medicine? They have made researchers look much harder at the lock-and-key effect. As a result, they learned that estrogen receptors may be different in different cells of the body; for example, the estrogen receptors on the breast and the uterus, two sites where we have long worried about cancer. It turns out that these receptors are quite different, so a SERM can be blocked from entering the breast or the uterus. More SERM-like products are in the pharmaceutical pipeline, and, of course, much more research needs to be done.

92 Can you please define the words that "SERM" is an acronym for?

SERM is an acronym for selective estrogen receptor modulator. Let's dissect those words and provide their meaning as they are used in the context of this new group of compounds.

Selective: acts only on certain body parts or in certain areas of the body.

Estrogen: the naturally occurring female hormone that is produced in a woman's ovaries. Estrogen acts on many areas throughout a woman's body.

Receptor: a specific site in a cell of the body, which can be turned on or off by a natural hormone or by a drug or compounded hormone or substance.

Turning on a receptor creates an action or a series of actions or effects.

Modulator: something that acts to regulate or activate something else.

This whole new class of compounds is going to add greatly to the other means available by which women can obtain more comprehensive health protection during menopause and the post-menopausal years.

93 What functions would the ideal SERM perform?

If medical science could bring us the ideal SERM, it would probably protect our bones, our breasts, our uterus, our heart, our brain, our skin, and every other place in our body that suffers or may in the future suffer from a lack of estrogen. It might, indeed, represent the magic bullet that we all seek. For me, it would turn off midlife weight gain and ensure that I never lost a single centimeter of my five-foot six-inch height. It would also permit me to look good in a bikini now and forever and to be in robust good health for as long as I lived.

I'm being facetious, of course, but I would happily settle for strong bones, heart, and brain throughout my life and protection from breast cancer. I would also like to remember the first and last names of everyone I meet, know exactly where I was heading when I began to speak, and know what I did with my car keys and sunglasses and whether I closed the garage door when I left home. This may all be possible.

94 I know that the Eli Lilly company engaged in studies of raloxifene and that their data suggest that this compound, which was under study for the prevention of osteoporosis, may go beyond that to offer a new choice of therapy for keeping postmenopausal women healthy. What did that data actually demonstrate?

The clinical trial results with raloxifene are very significant. They demonstrated that raloxifene, when compared with a calcium-supplemented placebo, prevented bone loss in the hip and spine. They showed that this compound increased bone mineral density by 2 to 3 percent in the hip, spine, and total body. This increase in bone mineral density — and that's what we all worry about losing — was significant at twelve months and remained in place at twenty-four months. The placebo group continued to lose bone mineral density throughout the entire twenty-four month period. This data has important implications for osteoporosis protection. After all, osteoporosis remains the number four killer of women — and is a preventable disease.

The effects of raloxifene on other organs of the body were also studied during the clinical trials. To study whether raloxifene would be cardioprotective, the effects of raloxifene on blood lipids and other indicators of risk for heart attacks and strokes were evaluated throughout the trials, which included a six-month study of 390 postmenopausal women. Raloxifene was shown to reduce LDL and total cholesterol, which when elevated are risk factors for hardening of the arteries and heart attacks, but not to alter HDL cholesterol or triglycerides. Furthermore, in the uterus, raloxifene did not stimulate growth of tissue or induce spotting or bleeding.

There is obviously more work to be done to perfect SERMs, but Evista (raloxifene) is the first real hope that women concerned about breast cancer have for relief of some of the serious long-term symptoms of menopause, such as osteoporosis. Recent important developments in SERM trials may mean that more highly refined SERMs with the ability to affect only specific receptor cells may be on the way over the next few years.

The data the FDA approved for raloxifene covered a two-year period during which about two thousand women took part in clinical trials focusing primarily on raloxifene as a drug for the prevention of osteoporosis. The FDA reviewed this new compound on what is termed a "priority review status." Raloxifene became available by prescription in January 1998. It is called Evista.

95 Are other SERMs in the FDA pipeline?

Other SERMs are currently under investigation in many places in the world, to learn of their potential role in treating advanced breast cancers. Pfizer Pharmaceutical is investigating the ability of droloxifene to slow cancerous breast cell growth. According to Allen Kraska, Ph.D., who heads up Pfizer's project, there is a chemical difference between tamoxifen, which has been in use for quite some time, and droloxifene. His research team is studying how and if droloxifene is safe in terms of protecting the uterus and whether it builds bone mass.

Another manufacturer is studying a SERM called idoxifene. We can be pretty certain that laboratories at various pharmaceutical companies throughout the world are working on other selective estrogen receptor modulators and that they are in the investigative pipeline. You can be sure that we will be hearing more and more about SERMs in the next few years.

96 So will SERMs replace HRT or ERT, or will they become an alternative choice?

Marla Ahlgrimm, R.Ph., president of Women's Health America, a compounding pharmacy, doesn't see SERMs as a replacement for estrogen. "SERMs can't take the place of the body's natural hormones. The hormone estradiol [estrogen] affects 300 to 400 sites in the body. SERMs are meant to act only in very specific places in the body." According to Elizabeth Barrett-Connor, M.D., professor and chief of the division of epidemiology at University of California at San Diego School of Medicine, viewing SERMs as an alternative to HRT is premature.

There is little doubt that the advent of SERMs is a major step forward in terms of postmenopausal women's health and another big gun in the arsenal to combat certain diseases. But we have to understand that like everything else available up to now, it's not going to be a perfect fit for every woman.

There are other important investigations under way that are exploring other benefits of SERMs for postmenopausal women. In January 1998, the Osteoporosis Prevention and Artery Effects of Tibolone (OPAL) study began. Supported by Organon Ltd., its purpose is to test the effects of tibolone, another SERM, on changes in carotid artery wall thickness, bone, and cardiovascular risk factors. There are ten centers involved in the trial, five in Europe and five in the United States. The trial is scheduled to conclude in September 2001. The principal investigator in the United States is Robert D. Langer, M.D., M.P.H., associate professor of family and preventive medicine at the University of California, San Diego (UCSD).

In late March 1998, Eli Lilly announced the initiation of a large, prospective clinical trial, entitled Raloxifene Use for the Heart (RUTH), to determine the ability of Evista to prevent heart attacks and heart-related deaths in postmenopausal women. The RUTH trial will involve twenty-five countries and approximately ten thousand postmenopausal women who are at risk of heart attack. This worldwide trial will last up to seven and a half years. The principal investigator is Dr. Elizabeth Barrett-Connor.

Then in May 1998 data from the ongoing Evista Osteoporosis Trials, reported at the American Society of Clinical Oncology meeting, demonstrated reductions of more than 50 percent in breast cancer incidence among women enrolled in the osteoporosis trials. There were actually two separate presentations of data. The first, by Steven R. Cummings, professor of medicine and epidemiology, University of California, San Francisco, analyzed 7,705 women involved in a single osteoporosis treatment study and showed a 70 percent reduction in the incidence of newly diagnosed invasive breast cancers over a follow-up period of thirty-three months. The second, a report from V. Craig Jordan, Ph.D., director, breast cancer research, Robert H. Lurie Cancer Center, Northwestern University, culled information on 10,553 postmenopausal women (including those in the Cummings study) across nine separate, placebo-controlled osteoporosis prevention and treatment studies. Jordan's report noted a 54 percent reduction in the incidence of newly diagnosed breast cancers during the same period.

What does all this mean? It means very encouraging news for postmenopausal women. And there is more going on that you need to know about. There is another study called the Multiple Outcomes of Raloxifene Evaluation (MORE) trial, which is designed to assess the ability of Evista to treat postmenopausal women with osteoporosis and to prevent fractures in women. Interim results from the MORE trial were presented on September 14, 1998, at the annual meeting of the European Congress on Osteoporosis in Berlin, Germany. They showed Evista reduced by about half the risk of new spinal fractures in postmenopausal women after two years of treatment. And there's even more. The National Surgical Adjuvant Breast and Bowel Project has announced plans to begin a new large-scale breast cancer prevention trial, called the STAR trial, which will be a double-blind (that means neither the participants nor the investigators know which person is receiving which drug) randomized study in which twenty-two thousand postmenopausal women at increased risk for breast cancer age thirty-five years old or older would be assigned to take either tamoxifen or raloxifene orally for five years. NSABP researchers estimate that more than three hundred institutions will participate in this trial throughout the United States, Canada, and Puerto Rico.

PART THREE

Phytoestrogens — The Plants and Other Alternatives

9

What Are Plant Estrogens?

NOW we're getting into the most confusing area of estrogen replacement therapy — phytoestrogens, which quite simply means plant estrogens. "Phyto" is the Greek word for plant. A discussion of pharmaceutical estrogens — or synthetic estrogens, as they are also called — versus plant estrogens can get really heated. The basis for the argument, as I have witnessed it, usually stems from the belief that "natural" treatments and therapies are better. Whatever "natural" means in this context. To avoid the argument and be fair and balanced, let's look at phytoestrogens as a "nonhormonal" way to manage menopause.

Phytoestrogens actually bear a very striking resemblance to human estrogen and often mimic how our own estrogen works in the body. It is said that phytoestrogens exist in more than three hundred plants, and they might work their wonders without negative side effects — if we were sure how much of which plant, or combination of plants, is enough to offset both short-term and long-term menopause symptoms and changes. Like pharmaceutical replacement estrogen, the plant compounds are structurally similar to human estrogen, and like estrogen, they seem to be able to target and enter a human estrogen receptor. Plant estrogens are far weaker than pharmaceutical estrogens. Yet for some women they offer complete relief from the nuisance symptoms of menopause.

Bit by bit, here and there, the scientific community around the world has begun to look seriously at phytoestrogens. Small yet important studies have been done with the wild yam, beginning around the middle of the twentieth century. In 1990 a report surfaced in the *British Medical Journal* in which Australian investigators described a phytoestrogenic experiment wherein twenty-five postmenopausal women consumed foods that contained an abundance of plant estrogens, such as soy flour and linseed, and demonstrated a low-level estrogen response, with milder hot flashes and a lifting of minor depression.

The studies thus far have been small, but the effects have been notable. That shouldn't be too surprising when we consider that digitalis, one of the most important heart medicines, is made from the foxglove plant and that plant-based pharmaceuticals are the source of some of our major medicines. We waste time when we try to defend phytochemical against pharmaceutical therapy or vice versa. Ideally, we should try to find what is best for women's long-term health.

The reason for the dichotomy between hormonal and non-hormonal therapy stems, I believe, from the fact that a large segment of the forty to fifty million women in midlife in the United States alone who could take pharmaceutical hormones have opted not to do so. The figures vary somewhat, but most sources indicate that around 80 percent of women are absolutely unwilling to take pharmaceutical estrogen or estrogen plus progestin, if their uterus is intact. Most of the women with whom I have talked at length indicate fear of breast cancer as their number one reason, with fear of other negative long-term effects on their bodies as second, and "I just don't like to take drugs" as third. Some of the women cite the bother of spotting, the nuisance of continuing to have periods, the discomfort of breast tenderness, and the annoyance of weight gain as other reasons for turning their thumbs down when it comes to HRT or ERT. Yet many of these women show varying degrees of interest in taking phytoestrogens. This is the result of a growing body of scientific evidence worldwide that suggests that the weak estrogens in plants may assist in managing the so-called nuisance symptoms of menopause — hot flashes, night sweats, insomnia, and vaginal dryness — and may also offer some long-term benefits to the skeletal and cardiovascular systems. Some epidemiological studies have indicated that populations, like the Japanese, who regularly consume foods that are high in phytoestrogens appear to have a significantly lower incidence of cardiovascular disease, breast cancer, and — a piece of interesting information for the man in your life — even prostate cancer.

Now these phyto, or plant, estrogens may be the choice of some women, but before you jump on the bandwagon there is a lot you need to know. As I've said repeatedly in the years I've been lecturing and giving workshops on menopause and osteoporosis, no matter whether you choose to use pharmaceuticals or plant estrogens, it is up to you to learn all you can about them and to know how much of what you should be taking. So let's spend some time with phytoestrogens.

97 How many classes, or types, of phytoestrogens are there?

Isoflavones, lignans, and *coumestans* are the three classes of phytoestrogens. Isoflavones are found in soybeans, lentils, and some other beans, like lima and kidney beans. Lignans are found in flaxseed, some grains, bread, vegetables, and fruits. Coumestans are found in seed sprouts, alfafa, and fodder crops. Most plants contain some phytoestrogens, but it is those in the classification of isoflavones that offer estrogenic activity most like human estrogen.

The major isoflavones are genistein, diadzein, and equol. The main lignans are enterolactone and enterodiol. We will not cover coumestans, because they are found primarily in animal feed. What we are discovering here as we go along is that diet plays a very vital role in our health before, at, and after menopause. A study published in the *British Medical Journal* described how adding more phytoestrogens to our diet can change how menopause affects us.

A new dietary supplement of natural estrogens for women

experiencing midlife changes called Promensil came on the market in mid-1998. Promensil, a product of Novogen, is derived from red clover, one of nature's richest sources of isoflavone plant estrogens. It can be found over-the-counter in most supermarkets, pharmacies, and health food stores and might be something you wish to consider if you are thinking about trying plant estrogens.

98 What are the best sources of isoflavones?

Soy, soy, soy. It seems that soy may turn out to be one of our magic bullets. Soy appears to diminish menopause symptoms and help to prevent osteoporosis, heart disease, and breast cancer, all at the same time. The Japanese diet is filled with soy, and Japanese women have a lower incidence of osteoporosis, heart disease, breast cancer, and hot flashes and night sweats than we do in the United States. All this seems to be related to their consuming large amounts of soy protein on a daily basis. There are a number of studies under way right now to learn the total effects of soy protein on the diet and to determine how much we require. Soybeans contain the two main isoflavones, genistein and diadzein.

Some studies have already suggested that just one serving of a soy food — eight ounces of soy milk or 1/2 cup of tofu — a day can lower your risk of some kinds of cancers. Wonderful claims are made for soy, but like those for vitamin E, many claims have not been studied rigorously or at all. Still it seems, inasmuch as the average Asian woman consumes about 100 milligrams more per day of soy than an American woman, who usually consumes only 1 to 3 milligrams per day, that we could safely increase our soy intake with no problems and probably with good results.

99 What are good sources of soy?

Fresh soybeans are an excellent source, but you can usually only find them in Asian grocery stores or on the menus of some Japanese restaurants. Fresh beans need to be boiled for ten or fifteen minutes before they are ready to eat. You can find canned, frozen, or dried soybeans in health food stores and Asian markets. Those stores also often carry soy nuts, soy milk, miso, tempeh, and tofu, products which are becoming more available in local supermarkets. Miso, most often used in soup, is a fermented soybean paste. Soy flour can be used in baking some items, but it doesn't work well in all recipes, so don't automatically assume that soy flour can replace wheat or other kinds of flour. Check it out carefully. There are now soy cookbooks in most bookstores. I consider tofu to be the most magical of all soy foods. It can be cut up into stir-fries, casseroles, salads, soups, and stews, and can even replace the sour cream on your baked potato. You can find tofu yogurt in supermarket freezers. Birds Eye has a new frozen product called Sweet Beans, which is frozen soybeans! Soy-protein powders, meant to be mixed with milk or juice, are a good choice, too; they make wonderful smoothies. Just make sure that the products you purchase contain soy protein isolate, which means the soy has not been washed in alcohol. (Some soy companies use an alcohol bath to get rid of soy's natural fat and sugar, and in the process wash away the isoflavones, which means your soy benefits have also disappeared.)

If soy is so wonderful, how much should you consume? That's the big question. A study is currently under way at Bowman-Gray School of Medicine in Winston-Salem in which women drink a soy beverage that contains 20 milligrams of isoflavones, and the effects are measured in an attempt to learn how much soy a postmenopausal woman should consume. Other studies report that you need a minimum of 20 grams of soy powder a day to subdue hot flashes and night sweats, and as much as 35 to 60 grams of soy protein to drop cholesterol levels and start to build bone. There is research under way in several places, but there are no concrete answers yet.

100 I keep hearing about the benefits of flaxseed oil. What is it?

Flaxseed oil is pressed from flaxseeds, which are loaded with lignans, one of the classes of phytoestrogens. It has been suggested that just one tablespoon of flaxseed oil is equivalent to a cup of soy milk. Interestingly, flaxseed has been shown to have similar benefits to soy, perhaps anticarcinogenic properties and the ability to stifle menopause symptoms as well. In an article entitled "The Role of Soy Products in Reducing Risk of Cancer" that appeared in the *Journal of the National Cancer Institute* July 1991, Mark Messina estimated that 200 milligrams of soy equals 0.3 milligram of pharmaceutical estrogen. That was the lowest dose in which pharmaceutical oral estrogen was available by prescription until Fempatch came along. I know this is a bit vague, but all I have been able to find are estimated amounts of phytoestrogens to compare with drugs. There are a number of books on using soy and flaxseed in the diet, such as *The Hot Flash Cookbook* listed in appendix B.

101 Are any herbs high in phytoestrogens?

A very limited amount of research has been done to show that the herbs taken by women, such as black cohosh, dong quai, and chasteberry, which are high in phytosterols (plant estrogens and progesterones in weak form) are useful in balancing hormones during the menopause transition. These herbs are used for medicinal purposes, and many prescription drugs are based on herbs that have proven safe and effective. Black cohosh, dong quai, and chasteberry can usually be found in health food stores. Black cohosh (*Cimicifuga racemosa*) root is the basis for a product called Remifemin, which comes in capsule form and is available over the counter in pharmacies. It is distributed in the U.S. by Enzymatic Therapy. Remifemin appears to decrease hot flashes, as well as to help with digestion, pelvic muscle strength, water retention, and nervousness. Dong quai (*Angelica sinensis*), included in many Chinese herbal formulas, has been used for years by women in the Far East to maintain appropriate levels of estrogen. Although its phytoestrogens are active, they are much less potent than estrogen. Herbalists often recommend dong quai to eliminate hot flashes and other menopause symptoms. Chasteberry (*Vitex agnus castij*) is an herb that is used to balance female hormones. It is said to work for PMS symptoms as well as for menopause symptoms; however, this gentle herb often takes several months before its positive effects are noticed.

All of these herbs can be taken in different forms, as an infusion or a tincture or sometimes brewed as a tea. But a word of caution is necessary here. Herbs can be toxic if ingested in the wrong quantities. You can also have an allergic reaction to herbs. You really need to learn as much as you can about an herb before using it, because you also want to make sure that it will not exacerbate other medical problems or symptoms you may be having.

It is interesting to note that a study of dong quai done by Bruce Ettinger, senior investigator, division of research, at Kaiser Permanente Laboratories in Oakland, California, demonstrated that dong quai when used alone was no better than a placebo in altering estrogen levels or in treating hot flashes or other menopause symptoms. People who understand Chinese medicine are quick to point out that dong quai is never used alone in Chinese herbal formulas. Yet women are buying it in health food stores and using it that way to try to combat the symptoms of menopause.

Another finding, reported in the abstract of the eighth annual meeting of the North American Menopause Society in 1997, concerned a ginseng extract called Ginsana. The report came from investigators in Sweden, where as many as 40 percent of women reported using herbal compounds to relieve menopause symptoms. The study found that Ginsana did enhance a sense of well-being and relieve some symptoms but that it did not help with vasomotor symptoms such as hot flashes.

In addition to the herbs mentioned, there are phytosterol creams made from yams and some soybean extracts that are applied on the body to diffuse menopausal symptoms but my questions always remain the same, "How much cream is enough? How much is too much? How do we know how much is absorbed? and Is the absorption rate constant?"

102 **If plant estrogens are weak to begin with will I destroy any of their value in cooking them?**

Lightly steaming most vegetables is a good, and tasty, idea. Don't worry about phytoestrogens losing their efficacy, even at temperatures ranging between 350 and 500 degrees.

103 **Should I take phytoestrogens?**

It's another choice that you have. At present, there is no concrete answer, although there are many such recommendations. I can't find research studies to bear out these recommendations scientifically, but I have heard much in the way of anecdotal evidence. Some women are enthusiastic about phytoestrogens not only because they have been satisfied with the results of using them, but also because they consider them to be "natural" treatments. Scientific validation is still lacking, but with the large number of studies on phytoestrogens being conducted in so many and varied places in the world, we will have better answers in the future.

104 **What are some foods that contain phytoestrogens?**

You probably consume many phytoestrogens without realizing their estrogenic value. See how many phytoestrogenic foods you consume regularly in this list:

apples
asparagus
barley
beans
blackberries
bok choy
carrots
cherries
corn
dried seaweed
fennel
flaxseed

garlic
grains
green pepper
hops
kale
licorice
milk
mustard greens
oats and oat bran
olive oil
onions
peas
pears
pomegranate
radishes
rice bran
rye
soy products
squash
sunflower seeds
wheat germ
yams

10

What Are Other Alternatives to Estrogen?

HE alternatives to ERT are many and varied. Certainly, nutritional supplements have much to offer women who cannot or choose not to use prescription hormones or phytoestrogens. There are also many therapies ranging from acupuncture to yoga that work well for many women. And a vast range of lifestyle improvements can reduce or eliminate the symptoms of menopause.

In fairness to yourself, you should check out these alternatives and see how and whether they work for you, or better yet, consider combining some with the pharmaceutical or plant estrogen that you are already using. That's what I do. I add vitamins and minerals to my daily regimen, I use acupuncture or acupressure massage, and I do yoga twice a week. I do other forms of exercise, have eliminated smoking (more than twenty-five years ago), and try to keep a healthful diet, basically eliminating excessive use of alcohol, salt, caffeine, colas, and protein, particularly from red meat.

In this chapter, let's review why vitamins and minerals, relaxation and other stress-reducing activities, and good nutrition and exercise can help to relieve menopause symptoms and enhance our health and longevity. A word of caution, though. If you want to experiment with vitamin and mineral supplements for symptom relief, take the time to read and learn about them, to understand their properties and what they might be able to do for you. It wouldn't hurt to discuss your thoughts with your physician or a qualified nutritionist. It is vitally important that you are taking the right dose, because overdosing on some vitamins and minerals can have toxic effects. In terms of vitamins and minerals, too much may be worse than too little.

105 Does vitamin E diminish or eliminate hot flashes and night sweats, and can I get it from foods?

Although there is no hard scientific evidence that it works, vitamin E is a staple for many women, offering them hot flash control as well as many other benefits. Vitamin E really works for me in that regard. When I was still in perimenopause and having those heat wave attacks, I took 800 International Units (IU) of vitamin E every day. I took 400 IU in the morning with my calcium-fortified orange juice and another 400 IU before bed to stop sweating at night. Vitamin E was first suggested to me by the owner of my neighborhood health food store, a man who knows a lot about what he sells. My doctor, although reminding me that there was no scientific proof of its effectiveness, agreed that I should try vitamin E. I have been on ERT for a number of years now, but I still take one 400 IU capsule of vitamin E each morning for its other properties and — this is important — if I am under a lot of stress and experience what I call break-through hot flashes, I double my dose of vitamin E and they disappear again.

In the past few years, more and more articles have appeared in major medical journals crediting vitamin E with maintaining our good health in many ways. In terms of treating the symptoms of menopause, in addition to stifling hot flashes vitamin E has shown real promise as a treatment for vaginal dryness and lifting mood. In treating vaginal atrophy (thinning and drying), some women use vitamin E topically with success, opening a capsule and applying the vitamin E oil directly on the vaginal tissues whenever they feel uncomfortable. Research studies over the last two decades have suggested that vitamin E may be helpful in improving some skin conditions, in treating osteoarthritis, and in preventing heart disease. But before you start taking vitamin E, check with your doctor; it is not usually recommended for anyone with a rheumatic heart condition, diabetes, or high blood pressure, and it should not be used at all by anyone taking digitalis. Megadoses of anything should be avoided or, at least, carefully considered. There has been some concern about too much vitamin E causing liver problems.

Vitamin E is available in some vegetable oils, seeds, raw nuts, and fruits and vegetables. The best sources are wheat germ (sprinkle some on your cereal), lettuce, and green peas. Other major food sources of vitamin E include asparagus, cucumber, and kale; oils made from wheat germ, soybean, sesame, corn, or safflower, and herring, mackerel, and haddock; lamb and liver (watch out for high cholesterol), brown rice, millet, and mangos. Vitamin E is destroyed by overzealous cooking, so to get the most out of vegetables loaded with vitamin E, if you must cook them at all then just lightly steam them.

In terms of using the oils mentioned above, recent research published in the *Archives of Internal Medicine,* January 12, 1998, suggests that the polyunsaturated fat in soybean, corn, and safflower oil may increase the risk of breast cancer. The study, done at the Karolinska Institute in Stockholm, was directed by Dr. Alicja Wolk and included 61,471 women. There was no doubt that the findings favored monounsaturated fats such as olive, canola, sunflower, and peanut oils.

This research is particularly compelling because it supports earlier investigations by scientists in the United States, Spain, Greece, and Italy that showed a link between olive oil and other sources of monounsaturated fats and a reduction in the risk of breast cancer. Although there is still debate about whether or not the Swedish study is conclusive, it does seem like a good idea to substitute olive, canola, sunflower, and peanut oil for other oils, shortenings, animal fats, and margarines in your diet, while limiting your total fat consumption. In countries that adhere to the

Mediterranean diet, where olive oil use is high, the incidence of heart disease is low.

106 I've heard that vitamin A is good for my skin. What are good sources of vitamin A?

Vitamin A is necessary for growth and maintenance of the mucous membranes, the eyes, and the skin. The U.S. recommended daily allowance for vitamin A (in the form of beta carotene) is 5,000 IU. Vitamin A can be found in large amounts in carrots, sweet potatoes, and yams, and in lesser amounts in pumpkin, broccoli, yellow squash, spinach, tomato, kale, cantaloupe, and mangos. Vitamin A is considered to be one of the antioxidant vitamins, which are discussed in the answer to question 108.

107 Will vitamin B_6 stop bloating?

Many women use it for that purpose, among other reasons. Vitamin B_6 (pyridoxine) in a small dose, such as 50 milligrams per day, can work as a natural diuretic. When it does, it is known to counteract the water retention that makes so many women using estrogen feel bloated and uncomfortable. There are other natural diuretics that may help as well, such as parsley, watercress, kelp, and cranberry juice. Be careful, though. Megadoses of vitamin B_6 can cause nerve damage. Yet a lack of B_6 can cause sleep problems and anxiety symptoms. The proper use of vitamin B_6 can be likened to the story of Goldilocks and the three bears. You've got to find the dose that is "just right" for you. Some food sources of vitamin B_6 are almonds, sesame seeds, pumpkin seeds, sunflower seeds, wheat germ, brown rice, rice bran, chicken, shrimp, salmon, tuna, and, of course, many vegetables, such as asparagus, broccoli, brussels sprouts, cauliflower, green peas, and sweet potatoes. Among its other values, vitamin B_6 is also known as a stress-buster.

108 What are antioxidants, and will they relieve menopause symptoms?

Antioxidants are believed to prevent cancer development by removing free radicals from our systems. Oxygen-free radicals are created during the oxidation process. Antioxidant protection is important because free radicals may damage our genetic material (DNA) and damaged genes can interfere with our cells' ability to halt cancerous changes. Free radicals may also oxidize proteins in the blood that carry cholesterol and thus be responsible for plaque buildup on the walls of arteries. Free radicals are a classification of chemicals. They may be viewed as loose cannons — harmful chemicals running around trying to land somewhere in our bodies and do some damage. Vitamins A, C, and E are considered to be antioxidants and should be taken together to function best in your system. These vitamins have demonstrated some protective effects against cancer cells' development in the breasts, lungs, colon, pancreas, and other important organs. Obviously, the protective effects of vitamin C on breast cancer in postmenopausal women is important. There have also been studies that suggest vitamin E reduces the risk of recurrence in women with stage II breast cancer. Vitamin E's help with hot flashes and vaginal dryness, both menopausal symptoms, was explained in the answer to question 105.

109 So should I start taking antioxidants?

It seems that using antioxidants might be a good idea, but if you do take supplements, don't go overboard. Studies are under way that look at the value of these antioxidants, and so far vitamin E is the only one demonstrating help in preventing cancer and heart disease. Earlier studies have actually been disappointing. So use caution. Take antioxidants in recommended doses only. They can be toxic at higher doses. Obtain your antioxidants from a reliable source and make sure you know what is in every pill that you take. Beware of unwanted additives. If you prefer, choose antioxidant food sources to help reduce the risk of cancer. Carrots, dark green leafy vegetables, and sweet potatoes are good sources. Notice here again the value of the sweet potato.

110 How much vitamin C should I take?

The current recommended daily allowance (RDA), about 40 milligrams per day, is probably way too low for vitamin C to do all its work. Two hundred milligrams may be the right dose, according to Dr. Mark Levine, chief of molecular and clinical nutrition at the National Institutes of Health (NIH). Also, 200 milligrams of vitamin C daily should be easily obtainable from foods, especially if you follow the most recent Department of Agriculture food chart, which tells us to eat five or more servings of fruits and vegetables each day. If you, like many Americans, are not consuming a diet rich in fruits and vegetables, you may need to consider taking a vitamin C supplement. If you do, it has been said that time-release vitamin C is best.

Vitamin C can be very helpful. Its anti-stress properties provide calming effects. It is said to prevent excessive menstrual bleeding, to thwart an oncoming cold if taken early enough, to help heal burns and wounds, and to maintain collagen, the main protein that supports our skin, tendons, cartilage, connective tissue, and bones. Vitamin C is easy to find in food. It is abundant in fruits such as oranges, cantaloupe, grapefruit, mango, papaya, and strawberries, to name just a few. Excellent vegetable sources are broccoli, brussels sprouts, cabbage, cauliflower, and most greens.

111 Can't I just get everything I need from a good multiple vitamin?

The answer to that question is another yes and no. A good multivitamin provides the RDA of most vitamins and minerals. So, yes, it is good to take one each day to be on the safe side, because all too often our jam-packed days don't allow for healthful eating. However, if you, like me, need additional amounts of various vitamins and minerals, you have to take them along with your multivitamin. For example, as well as my multivitamin, I take ginkgo, extra vitamin E — 400 IUs — and extra calcium that contains magnesium and vitamin D. I also take one ibuprofen tablet per day, because studies show some possible effectiveness in protection against Alzheimer's disease, and one baby aspirin at bedtime every other day to protect against heart disease. All of the above is in addition to my daily ERT. I'm hedging my bets, and I feel great!

112 What other herbs are used to suppress menopausal symptoms?

Besides the ones I discussed in the answer to question 101, there are a number of herbs that when taken in moderation may alleviate some symptoms in some women. Today, St. John's wort heads the popularity list. It is said that it can be used successfully for hormonal or minor depression, anxiety, mood swings, and the like. It has even been called the modern woman's answer to Prozac, but studies have yet to confirm that. Evening primrose oil, ginseng, licorice root, chamomile, passionflower, and blackberry root have long been on the list. They may work because these plants contain estrogen — actually phytoestrogen, as described in chapter 9. Here again, let caution be your watchword. Herbs can be toxic if ingested in too large a quantity and may also cause an allergic reaction. Yet herbs can also do wonderful things. Take ginseng, for example. Here is a plant estrogen that can improve energy and may also relieve hot flashes. Yet I have not heard from a single woman that her physician suggested she try ginseng. That is because to suggest it would be like prescribing estrogen without knowing how much the patient is ingesting. So, if you would like to sip ginseng tea to treat menopausal symptoms, be sure to find out how much to sip each day.

Other herbs rich in phytosterols (plant estrogens and progesterones) that may work to balance hormones during the menopause transition include black cohosh, dong quai, and chasteberry. Again, these are weaker than pharmaceutical estrogens and a greater amount is required to have the desired effect. Caution is required here, too. Learn the properties of herbs before you begin taking them, to assure that you are taking the right amount. Susun S. Weed, author of *Menopausal Years,* says, "Using plants rich in phytosterols is remarkably different from taking hormones. Phytosterols provide hormonal building blocks rather than the hormones themselves, allowing your body to create the precise amounts and combination of the hormones needed." That's good, but I ask, how much of what does the job?

Chamomile is another helpful herb. Since insomnia is high on the symptom list of many women who filled out my questionnaires or who have contacted me, I have asked them to share with my readers what worked for them. Of course, the number one insomnia squelcher is estrogen, but many women say herbal teas containing chamomile, catnip, valerian root, or passionflower helped them enormously. Other women suggest long evening walks, warm baths, or a glass of wine or warm milk before bed.

Women who seek symptom relief with herbs often tell me that they are a bit confused and scared initially. One of their more pressing questions usually deals with wanting to know what is "a tincture" and what is "an infusion." I know how they feel. Just walking into a health food store can be confusing, and looking at shelf after shelf of products I know little about is frightening. Let's try to clear up the nomenclature a bit. A tincture refers to fresh plant material that has been steeped in either alcohol or vinegar. The alcohol tincture usually keeps a bit longer, but is not good for women with an allergy or an aversion to alcohol. (Is this Lydia Pinkham's Vegetable Compound reinvented?) All kinds of tinctures are available and the products have a long shelf life. An infusion is something else again. It is usually prepared by taking an ounce or more of fresh or dried plant material and steeping it in a quart of boiled water for several hours. The resulting infusion must be refrigerated in order to last for a few days.

113 Will Chinese medicine make the menopause transition smoother?

Chinese medicine has been very helpful to women who either cannot or choose not to take estrogen and yet are suffering with menopausal symptoms. Some Chinese herbs, such as dong quai and ginseng, have already been mentioned, but there is much more to Chinese medicine than herbs. Acupuncture, an ancient Far Eastern healing art, has been very successful in symptom relief. It involves the insertion of incredibly thin needles just under the skin at certain points on the body's "meridians" for the purpose of unblocking energy, or *qi* (pronounced chee). If you wish to explore this excellent form of therapy, be sure that the therapist is licensed and uses disposable needles. As with any medical service, check the practitioner's credentials carefully. My own licensed acupuncturist, Kristen Lee, in Del Mar, California, has explained to me the theory in Chinese medicine in regard to menopause. She told me that the feelings of unrest and irritability, and even hot flashes and night sweats, are considered in Chinese medicine to be manifestations of a kidney/liver "yin" deficiency and the consequent flaring of Fire. I must admit I don't completely understand the wonders of Chinese medicine, yet women tell me that acupuncture coupled with one or more Chinese herbal formulas can often work wonders in dealing with these problems. For more information about acupuncture, contact the American Association of Acupuncture and Oriental Medicine, which is listed in appendix D.

114 Can you take too many vitamins and minerals?

More vitamins and minerals is not necessarily better than less. Spend some time learning about vitamins and minerals and what they can do to help you become healthier and stronger. Remember, megadoses of anything are not good, so before you increase the amounts of what you are using, discuss it with your physician. If he/she is not a vitamin-mineral proponent, and most physicians are not, then talk to your pharmacist. I often get my most valuable information from mine.

115 Is alternative medicine a trend or is it here to stay?

In the *New England Journal of Medicine* in 1993, David Eisenberg, M.D., and his colleagues documented how popular alternative medicine is with health care consumers. Dr. Eisenberg, director of the center for Alternative Medicine at Beth Israel Medical Center in Boston, estimated that in 1990 some sixty million Americans were using some form of alternative medicine and making 425 million visits to alternative medicine practitioners. That number represents more visits to alternative healers than to conventional physicians, which numbered 388 million visits that same year.

The problems with ignoring conventional medical interventions is that you might miss something important. So it is vital that you share with your physician the facts about your alternative medical therapies. It seems that it is up to us, the patients — the consumers of health and medical care — to surround ourselves with the best in both conventional and alternative medicine. We have to be aware of the fact that the very nature of what we call alternative medicine indicates that whatever it is, it is not taught in medical schools. Therefore, your medical doctor is generally unaware of most alternative therapies and remains skeptical. Nonetheless, it is up to us to face her or him with our symptoms and our choices of therapies. Only then can we integrate the best in alternative medicine with the best in conventional medicine to assure ourselves the best medical care. Then we can benefit from the best in "integrative medicine." The interest in alternative medicine continues unabated, but we must be careful not to throw away all that is good and proven in conventional medicine in our haste to take control of our health and our health care.

11

What Lifestyle Changes Should I Make?

CHANGE of life, as menopause has so unfortunately been labeled, is not what menopause is about, unless you take it quite literally to mean — change of lifestyle. What I am proposing here is that women take an active role at menopause, rather than passively permitting some biological changes to diminish their quality of life. The debate for us should not be whether menopause is or is not an estrogen deficiency disease. Menopause is not a *disease* of any sort. The debate for us should also not be solely whether we wish to take estrogen or not. That's not our number one challenge either. The debate we should be having with ourselves is whether or not we are doing everything we can to improve our midlife health by improving our lifestyle.

Quite frankly, I see exercise as the elixir of life. I have seen women, and men for that matter, totally change physically, mentally, and socially when they begin a solid exercise program. It's not only those happy endorphin hormones that begin to circulate, it is also that mentally uplifting feeling of taking charge that permeates their entire being. There is nothing more important than being in control of your body and, thus, of your life.

Year after year, study after study shows the value of exercise. It helps to prevent heart attack and stroke; and a report from the American Heart Association in late 1997 showed a relationship between exercise and the prevention of breast cancer. One of the findings of the Harvard Nurses' Health Study, as reported in the *New England Journal of Medicine* in 1995, was that women who gain weight between the ages of thirty and fifty encounter the biggest risk factor for breast cancer later in life. There are still many debates concerning health, but whether or not you need to exercise is not one of them. Sadly, fewer than 30 percent of the American population exercises with any regularity. If you could improve your health and change the course of your life, would you? If your answer is yes, then begin exercising today. You can begin with something as simple as a walk around the block.

Throughout her younger life, but most important from the perimenopausal to the postmenopausal years, exercising may be the most important thing a woman can do for her physical and mental health. With or without estrogen therapy, exercise is important; it protects against heart disease, osteoporosis, some forms of cancer, and weight gain. Interestingly, although not surprisingly, weight gain is the challenge women complain about the most. The answer to weight gain probably is, in large part, exercise. Exercise can also alleviate many menopausal symptoms, including hot flashes, night sweats, insomnia, and difficulties with digestion. Exercise revs up blood circulation, and as more blood reaches the brain and the endorphin hormones are released women generally feel better — more alert and happier.

Exercise is but one factor in promoting good health. Others include the need to eat healthful meals in the proper proportions, to stop smoking, and to cut back or eliminate other harmful substances such as alcohol and caffeine. It is also vital to reduce negative stresses in our lives.

116 What is the difference between aerobic and anaerobic exercise?

Let's start with the basic meaning of the word aerobic, which comes from the Greek word for air. That makes it easy to remember that the type of exercise that depends on air, or breathing, is aerobic. The type of exercise that does not depend on air is anaerobic. We need both kinds. Aerobic exercise works with your breathing to deliver oxygen to the muscles of the body. It is vital for cardiovascular health.

Anaerobic exercise helps to build muscle mass, strength, and flexibility. A good example of an anaerobic exercise is weight training. Aerobic exercise has its greatest effects on the cardiovascular system and on weight loss or weight maintenance. However, it is the conversion of fat to muscle mass that is achieved in anaerobic weight training that helps to burn more calories.

117 What kinds of exercise do women at menopause need?

Women at any age really need three kinds of exercise. We need stretching for flexibility, aerobic exercise to protect our hearts, and weight-bearing exercise to protect our bones and help ward off osteoporosis. Touching base with your physician if you have not been a regular exerciser is always a good idea before beginning a rigorous program.

When you set up your exercise program, it is important that you include the following elements: Start with an aerobic warm-up of a least six minutes. Then begin the exercise portion, which can be aerobic or anaerobic depending on what you are doing that day — for example, treadmill, or weight training — which should last for at least thirty minutes. Finally, allow time for a cool-down period of not fewer than five minutes, which should include a gradual lessening of intensity of your exercise activity, followed by stretching. Ideally, we should all try to get some aerobic exercise every day and do weight training two or three times a week on nonconsecutive days. If your time does not permit a daily cardiovascular aerobic workout, try to make sure you do cardio exercise at least three times a week for no fewer than thirty minutes.

118 How do I find my target heart rate, and do I need to monitor it in all kinds of exercise?

When you are working aerobically you should be working at your target heart rate. To determine that rate, subtract your age from 220, then figure 60 to 80 percent of that number as the range in which you can safely work. For example, if you are a fifty-year-old woman your maximum exercise heart rate, working at 100 percent, would be 170 beats per minute. How did I get the 170? By subtracting 50 (your age) from 220. Now take 60 percent of that number (170) and then 80 percent of it. When you do you learn that you can work between 102 and 136 heartbeats per minute. For best results, you must always work within your target heart rate range.

When you are exercising aerobically, check your heart rate by either counting the pulse beats in your neck or at your wrist for ten seconds and then multiply by six, or use one of the heart monitoring belts that encircle your chest. It's a good idea to check your heart rate periodically while you exercise, to make sure you're doing enough but not too much. If you are working out in a gym or have your own aerobic equipment at home you can monitor your heart rate by holding on to the sensors and checking the number on the electronic display.

119 How often must I exercise during menopause?

It's not just at menopause, it is throughout the rest of your life that you should exercise at least three times a week. Five times a week is even better. Try to pick exercise activities that you really enjoy; having fun is more than half the exercise battle. I read a couple of recent studies that demonstrated that we can divide up our exercise time periods and still derive significant benefits. For example, if you simply don't have a thirty-minute stretch of time, try exercising for three ten-minute periods during the course of the day. It is important that you get your heart rate into its target range for those ten minutes to derive the most benefit.

A large part of the problem in getting people to exercise in the past has been the length of time and the lists of the kinds of exercise activities that were deemed worthwhile. Only recently have gardening and heavy housework been included in calorie counts and have benefits been demonstrated from frequent short exercise periods. This newer approach to daily exercise certainly should encourage more women and men to exercise.

120 Is walking good enough exercise for me?

Walking is the most popular exercise in America and a good choice as a weight-bearing activity. There are now more than seventy million exercise walkers in the United States alone. Walking requires no equipment and only a good pair of walking shoes. What you wear with the shoes depends on your comfort and the weather. Do stretch before and after. A good smooth stretch — no bouncing — of your Achilles tendons and calves, your quadriceps, and your hamstrings is essential.

The consensus seems to be that walking for thirty to forty-five minutes per day at a pace of between three and three and a half miles per hour brings beneficial results. The only problem with walking seems to be that some women find it to be lonely. Others claim they intend to go walking but something always keeps them from it. Here are a number of ideas for getting going.

- Have a destination in mind. To keep on track, many people need to know where they're going.
- Plan to meet a friend at a specific time and use the half hour or forty-five minutes to walk and talk, forgoing a long telephone conversation and catching up on the news while getting your weight-bearing exercise accomplished.
- Become a nature buff and walk to watch the seasons change, noting budding trees, shrubs, flowers, and wildlife.
- Join a walking group or club, one that fines you when you've been a no-show, if you can find one.

- Walk at a mall and window shop while walking, but don't stop to buy anything.
- Use your Walkman to listen to music or a good audio book.
- Walk to the shops, to work, or to a friend's home instead of driving, if distance and safety permit.
- Park your car in the farthest spot from where you're going and walk to and from the car.
- Add some hilly areas to your walking route for extra effort.
- Use stairs instead of elevators, and walk up escalators.
- Keep a walking journal and review your progress periodically. Every once in a while reward yourself for a job well done.
- Learn to enjoy walking. It's our number one weight-bearing exercise.

121 What are you doing when you perform weight-bearing exercise, and which ones are best?

When you perform weight-bearing exercises you are actually stressing bone, and stressed bone builds, or replenishes, itself. The National Osteoporosis Foundation lists the following as preferred weight-bearing exercises: walking, stair climbing, hiking, jogging, treadmill, skiing (both downhill and cross-country), low-impact aerobic dance, dancing, and weight training either with weight machines like Nautilus or with free weights.

Other suitable lower-impact weight-bearing exercises include cross-country ski machines, stair-climbing machines, stair-stepping machines, and water aerobics. Note that swimming is not a weight-bearing exercise, so although it provides flexibility and some cardiovascular benefit, it does not help to maintain bone mass. If you like water exercise, perhaps you could swim and then do water aerobics, water walking, or water jogging to incorporate all three kinds of required exercise in a water program. In the last few years, a whole line of water exercise gear came on the market. There are wonderful water exercise belts that keep you buoyant while you water jog, and webbed, weighted gloves and footwear that offer added resistance.

122 **If I have never done so before, should I begin to lift weights now that I'm going through menopause?**

Lifting light weights is a good idea at any age. If you've never done this before, and if you have any kind of medical problem, discuss it with your physician. If you're gung-ho to get started, learn how to lift weights properly from a certified trainer or an exercise physiologist. This is not someone that you need to keep on your payroll for long, just long enough to develop your individualized weight-training program and to make sure you know exactly what you are doing. There are various ways to lift weights, either by machine, by hand-held weights, or with wrapped wrist and ankle weights. Start slowly and with light weights. You will usually be instructed to repeat each lift six to twelve times, at 60 to 80 percent of your maximum strength. This will improve muscle strength and muscle endurance and will protect your bones. Get comfortable and strong at each lifting level before you increase the weights, and add more weight slowly to avoid injury.

It is interesting to note that weight-training programs begun very late in life with senior adults have shown benefit. William Evans, director of the physiology laboratory at the Human Nutrition Research Center on Aging at Tufts University, co-authored a 1990 study showing that "nine men and women between the ages of eighty-seven and ninety-six increased the strength in the front of their thigh muscles by an average of 175 percent after eight weeks of supervised weight-lifting." Similar late-life workout studies done at Leisure World, a retirement community in southern California, and at New York University School of Medicine also demonstrated that exercise is beneficial and can increase muscle mass, build small amounts of bone, and enhance the health and well-being of senior adults. Other studies have shown similar results. It's never too late to begin.

A comprehensive weight-training program should be well balanced and designed to strengthen all major muscle groups—arms, shoulders, chest, back, abdomen, hips, and legs. If you plan to lift weights twice a week, don't do it on consecutive days. Alternate lifting with aerobic activities to give your muscles a chance to recover.

123 Does weight training burn calories?

Since avoiding weight gain is most women's greatest concern at midlife, consider this: twenty to thirty minutes of a weight-lifting workout will typically burn between 200 and 300 calories, depending on your existing muscle mass and degree of effort. And you will increase your muscle mass. That's important because every pound of additional muscle will burn an extra 30 to 50 calories a day.

According to the American College of Sports Medicine Guidelines, you need only add weight training to your exercise regimen twice a week. The Guidelines suggest performing three aerobic and two weight-training workouts each week, each workout to begin and end with five to ten minutes of stretching. If you are in good health, this is an excellent way to prevent osteoporosis as well as feel strong and in control, and to look good.

124 I am going through menopause and gaining weight. How do I stop this?

That's the midlife woman's major concern. Many women tell me they wish they had known this was going to happen when they were younger so they could have worked to avoid it. Actually, metabolism begins its slow and steady decline of between 1/2 and 1 percent per year when women are around the age of thirty-five. For some women the decline is so slow it is barely noticeable until around age fifty, when she typically swings through menopause. Let's say that a woman loses 1 percent of her metabolic burn per year from age thirty-five to age fifty. That's a 15 percent slowdown. And let's say that she neither decreases food intake nor increases exercise. That metabolic slowdown with nothing to offset it is the weight gain culprit for most midlife women.

The answer to weight gain is to establish sound, balanced, healthful eating and, of course, a well designed regular exercise program. We've already covered exercise, so let's stick with nutrition here. Most of us are aware that we need to follow a low-fat, calcium-rich, high-fiber diet. What does that mean? It means that by scanning the newest food pyramid developed by the U.S. Department of Agriculture we know that we need five to six serving of fruits and vegetables each day, lots of whole grains, and less protein and fat than we ever imagined.

125 How can I balance all the nutrients I need?

Balancing all of this is a real challenge. It means keeping fat intake between twenty and thirty grams per day. Don't cut out more fat than that unless instructed by your physician for other medical problems, because your skin, nails, and hair will suffer. Also, a little fat helps insulate our bodies against the cold. Balancing also means taking in at least 1,000 milligrams of calcium each day before menopause and upping that to 1,500 milligrams per day at menopause, if you are not taking estrogen. If you are on ERT or HRT, you can stay at 1,000 milligrams per day until age sixty-five, when it is recommended that all women and men increase their calcium intake to 1,500 milligrams per day.

Further, balancing means following the American Institute for Cancer Research's recommendation that we take in between twenty and thirty-five grams of fiber each day. Always increase fiber intake slowly to avoid digestion problems and remain socially acceptable. Don't go overboard on fiber either, because it can whisk away the vitamins and minerals in our system that we need.

The fat-free labels on food products have misled us, because often the fat that the product has been freed from has been replaced by sugar, which will turn into fat once inside your body. And we tend to eat more of a fat-free item. If a cookie is fat free, why not have three? Think of "fat free" as a label only for fruits and vegetables, whole grains, and beans, and not for packaged products. Also apply the "fat-free" label to the eight 8-ounce glasses of water you need to drink each day.

Watching your weight is really about balance. It's about eating the right foods and about eating less and exercising more. A whole category of cookbooks for women at and beyond menopause has appeared in recent years and bears looking into. Authors have attempted to provide recipes for the kind of eating we need to do to give us increased energy and more of the nutrients we require while taking in fewer calories.

126 Should I give up alcohol?

Not necessarily, but you should use it with moderation. It's confusing when we read that alcohol can benefit our heart but can also damage our liver and our pancreas and can be involved in certain kinds of cancer. Moderate use of alcohol means one drink a day, which may be in the form of a twelve-ounce can or bottle of beer, a four-ounce glass of wine, or one ounce of liquor. For women, that amount may be okay for helping to decrease heart disease. But a Harvard study reported in the July/August 1997 issue of *Menopause Management* hinted at increased risk of breast cancer when alcohol and estrogen interact. The study was small, only twenty-four women, half of them taking estradiol, and revealed increased estradiol levels in women on ERT after they had consumed very small amounts of alcoholic beverages. The more alcohol consumed, the more the levels rose. Not enough is known about the alcohol-estradiol connection, and you can be sure it is a subject for more investigation.

127 How do I reduce the stress in my life?

Stress is part of living. Some stresses are positive, some negative. Positive stresses are those which enable us to reach our life's goals. What you want to do is reduce the negative stresses, which are those extraordinary demands put upon us to which our minds and bodies must respond. The menopause time of life is filled with negative stress. We see and feel personal physical changes, and while we are trying to adapt to them we must often cope with critical family situations. The illness or loss of parents occurs around the time of our menopause, our nests empty of children, or our grown children return home with problems and sometimes with their own children. The menopausal woman is often said to be in the "sandwich generation," with stressful demands from the generation above and the generation below. And sometimes there is an even more painful push. Many women share stories of being replaced by the "trophy wife" that their mate feels he deserves because of his success or needs because he is feeling his own mortality. It is often hard to deal with the nameless and shameless terror that some men feel when they realize that they are aging, too. Frequently it is the attention of hard-bodied women young enough to be their daughters that momentarily erases their fears. So wonderful and talented wives who have spent their years aging companionably alongside their husbands are cast aside for no real reason, other than as one executive explained to his perfectly lovely and talented wife as he walked out the door, "When I'm with you I feel old!" Even if you are not the wife left behind, you can be faced with the child brides of your husband's friends as dinner companions.

The worst stress buildup comes from not dealing directly with stress. Recognize negative stresses in your life. Make a comprehensive list of what is bothering you and then prune it by eliminating what you can. If you are overcommitted at home or at work, look for ways to unload some things. Extend a deadline, drop a project, delay plans for a party, disinvite guests — do whatever you have to do to free some time for yourself. Try to clearly identify the sources of your stress and make a plan for avoiding or overcoming them. If you need outside help, see a counselor or therapist. It is best to discuss problems with a trained outside observer, for when you do you often come up with your own best solutions. The cost of therapy pales beside the ultimate cost to your health of unrelieved stress.

There are many ways to begin to eliminate stresses. For example, if you are constantly concerned because you are habitually late, give yourself more time by getting up earlier, getting ready sooner, or getting wherever you need to be earlier. If you have friends or family members that are problems for you, try to speak to them less frequently or avoid them altogether if you can.

Learn the three-deep-breaths routine and use it whenever you are in a stressful situation: Draw a deep breath in through your nose for a count of four, and let it out through your mouth for a count of six. Do that three times whenever you are faced with stress, and you will experience an automatic relaxation response, enabling you to switch from high to low gear. I find that after a month of using this stress-busting technique I have achieved some real relief from negative stresses. This type of controlled breathing when continued uninterrupted for five minutes or longer has actually been shown to reduce blood pressure by ten or eleven points.

128 What are some other sources of mind-body healing and relaxation?

Remember, nothing works for everyone. You need to experiment to find out what works best for you. Here's a rundown of techniques from which you can choose.

Relaxation therapy can help to relieve both stress and tension and in that way, with or without estrogen, help to minimize menopause symptoms. This technique involves a process through which you systematically relax from toes to head by consciously moving up your body, concentrating on and relaxing each part. Try it. Lie down in a darkened room. Close your eyes. Let your concentration begin at your toes, and tell them to relax. Next relax your ankles, your calves, knees, thighs, hips, and so on. By the time you reach your head, jaws, and eyes, you should be deeply relaxed. Lie still and enjoy the feeling for as long as you are able, and revisit it often.

Visualization is a very interesting technique. It is one in which you see yourself in an environment that you have created. For example, you are faced with another night of insomnia, so you visualize yourself lying on a beach, listening to the waves and feeling the sun beat down on you. You are warm, you are comfortable. Suddenly you feel happy, loved, and cozily enveloped by nature. Now you can sleep.

Biofeedback is another fascinating relaxation technique. It requires you to be hooked up to a piece of equipment that can help you train your mind to take control of your own heart rate, muscle tension, and even the temperature of your skin, all of which are the body's automatic responses. The feedback you are seeking may let you know when you have controlled your hot flashes, lowered your blood pressure, or even lowered your skin temperature. It comes from the equipment's readouts or sounds, which tell you whether you have succeeded in affecting whatever system you are trying to control.

Meditation is very helpful. I know people who take time to meditate for fifteen minutes morning and evening. They claim vastly improved mental and physical health.

Yoga combines physical exercise and meditation with deep breathing, permitting you to focus your attention and calm your mind. Yoga can also enhance joint and muscle strength and flexibility and help to maintain healthy bones. Like all the other relaxation therapies it may be useful in stemming the symptoms of menopause and the problems of aging. *Yoga Basics,* by Mara Carrico and the editors of *Yoga Journal,* can teach you to practice yoga in your own home. Mara Carrico has been teaching yoga for more than a quarter of a century and is the choreographer of *Jane Fonda's Yoga Exercise Workout* video.

Tai chi, an ancient Chinese discipline of fluid movement, can promote good health in many ways. It is known to improve flexibility, strength, and balance, promote a sense of well-being, and increase aerobic capacity as well. This is a no-impact exercise form that increases awareness and alertness yet is easy on muscles and bones. Well suited for all ages, tai chi is particularly helpful to older persons and those with arthritis, since it offers exercise without impact on the joints of the body. The only way to learn tai chi is from an experienced teacher. Qi gong is the primary Eastern exercise form that focuses on mind and body, offering an internal, contemplative state of being coupled with outward slow, focused movements that reward you with a deep sense of relaxation.

129 Will massage alleviate menopausal symptoms?

All kinds of massage can elicit calm and bring relief from the symptoms of menopause, particularly joint pain. There are many kinds of massage to try, but make sure you are working with a licensed massage therapist. Acupressure massage, like acupuncture itself, involves using digital pressure in the same spots on the meridians of the body in which needles would be inserted if you were having acupuncture. The purpose of this type of massage is to unblock the body's energies by relieving trigger points in the muscles. Acupressure is a deep form of massage. Shiatsu massage also works deep within the body. Swedish massage is usually a lighter and a more soothing massage. Foot reflexology involves working only on the feet, which, because there are corresponding points to all areas and organs of the body located on them, can be used to relax the entire body. There are other kinds of massage that work well, too. Explore, experiment, and see what works best for you. Live your life to the fullest.

12

Is Menopause Experienced the Same Way Throughout the World?

WAS giving a talk to the Las Vegas Medical Society, on the 104th floor of the Stratosphere Hotel the week it opened in 1997, about "Women's Perspectives of HRT." Following my talk there was a question-and-answer period, during which a young Asian gynecology resident asked the question that I have come to expect at some point in a gathering such as this. "How come," he asked, "American women make such a big deal about menopause, and it is hardly noticed by women in Japan?"

I had done my homework and I knew that there is no word for hot flash in the Japanese language. I also knew that the major menopause complaint of Japanese women is stiff shoulders. Only headaches ranked as a symptom for discussion, with about 28 percent of Japanese women experiencing them. Fewer than 10 percent of Japanese women experienced the nameless hot flashes, and just over 3 percent had night sweats. I also knew that Japanese women do not head for their trusty gynecologist with any symptoms, no matter what they are called. Typically, they appear to believe that the symptoms are natural and transitory. How then do we really know their collective menopause experience?

Japanese women have a life span of about eighty-two years,

and during the latter part of that span they develop osteoporosis twice as often as Japanese men, but less than half as frequently as Western women. Also, Japanese women develop osteoporosis later, in their seventies and eighties, while Western women are often faced with it in their fifties and sixties or even younger. Japanese women experience about one fourth the incidence of heart disease and breast cancer of American women. So what's going on here?

Does the explanation lie within their diet, which contains a lot of soy and soy products, a diet that has been in use generation after generation? Is it the fact that Japanese women exercise throughout their lives, walking everywhere? Does it have to do with the fact that they rarely drink alcohol or smoke? Although the answers to those questions have not been fully found through the scientific method, the odds are that each of those facts along with their genetic makeup in general account for the differences. Yet just a couple of years ago, when the Japanese Menopause Society was formed, Japanese women, learning of some of the antiaging benefits of estrogen, began to consider ERT and HRT. Interesting!

Mayan Indian women pass through menopause symptom free and also have no word for hot flashes. (In the United States, 75 to 85 percent of women experience hot flashes.) The Rajput women of India also are said to experience no hot flashes, and they view menopause as a graduation from pregnancy and parenting into a position of respect and dominance. Native American women are respected as wise elders and leaders within their tribes once they pass through menopause.

A fascinating study of the Hadza people of northern Tanzania was reported in the *New York Times,* September 16, 1997. This small group of 750 hunter-gatherers live today as their ancestors did, eschewing a modern lifestyle. The study, by Dr. Kristen Hawkes and her group at the University of Utah, found that Hadza women beginning in their fifties and into old age are viewed as among the most industrious members of their group and of invaluable assistance to younger members.

It may be that women in countries like Japan, where the diet is very high in phytoestrogens, simply have fewer hot flashes than women in other countries. That, however, is pure speculation. It also may be that in cultures where aging is rewarded women don't view menopause and hot flashes as problems but rather as signs that their good times are coming. The question is always raised as to whether some women make too big a deal of menopause symptoms, but as one woman who was nearly rendered nonfunctional until I began taking estrogen, I can tell you my perceptions were all in order. It was my symptoms that were extraordinary and debilitating.

It remains true in the United States that aging is not rewarded and that the menopausal woman is still faced with advertisements and images of the very young, very shapely, and very beautiful. Movie roles for middle-age women remain rare, although men are accepted as lovers until they're in their dotage.

130 Does the ginseng used by Chinese women account for their lack of hot flashes?

Who knows? Nothing in Western scientific literature proves that ginseng relieves hot flashes, but there is much evidence that it works. The Chinese have been using ginseng for more than three thousand years. Reports from China are anecdotal rather than the result of the rigorous investigations we might like. If you decide to use ginseng tea to relieve hot flashes, consult a Chinese medicine practitioner or someone reliable at your local health food store to learn about the quality of the product and how much you should be taking.

131 Are difficulties with menopause symptoms solely the province of American women?

Not at all. The truth is that women in many African tribes report problems with menopause that are very similar to those of Western women. European women have roughly the same experiences as American women, 15 percent of them sailing through menopause, or so they think (not knowing the quality of their bones), 15 percent having debilitating symptoms, as I did, and the remaining 70 percent ranging all over the board from minor to major problems with menopause symptoms.

Different cultures not only react differently to menopause but also appear to have different concerns about it. One study shows that Jews of European ancestry have menopause symptoms similar to American women while Jews from North Africa who live in Israel report few symptoms. Near Eastern Jews greatly fear a decline in their physical health while European Jews and other women in Europe are most concerned about decline in their mental health. Other women in various parts of the world are concerned first and foremost about their lack of fertility and desirability. It's a mixed bag of supercharged emotions.

132 Are there parts of the world where women gain status and additional freedom once they have become postmenopausal?

Much has been studied and written about cultural differences as we age. It is most interesting that, while in Western culture menopause may still be equated with aging and a lessening of powers, sexual and otherwise, in other cultures women soar after menopause. Women who have had their faces veiled throughout their youth and childbearing years are free to remove their veils. They are no longer segregated during monthly periods. They can join in activities with men and are free to travel. In many cultures they are included in the body politic. Indian women, women in Mexico, and the Cree women of western Saskatchewan may not begin to exercise their healing powers until they are past menopause. Tonganese women past menopause can engage in business and eat previously prohibited foods. Many native women may become matchmakers and midwives only after menopause. Other groups of women, such as Papuan women and some Chinese women, are freed from the power of their husbands once they are postmenopausal.

133 What do all these cultural differences mean?

They may suggest genetic or environmental differences. They may mean that menopausal symptoms are welcomed when women know that restrictions on their lives will soon be removed, and that the postmenopause can be a vital, rewarding time of life.

It wasn't too long ago that postmenopausal women in the United States and elsewhere were treated as old people. They even thought of themselves as old and somehow deserving of the "miseries" of old age. This has all changed, and menopause, once a taboo subject, is now out in the open. Women want answers to their questions. They want to feel better. This openness about menopause and the issues and symptoms surrounding it is only a development of the last decade. Women's advocates moved slowly and steadily toward gaining better information and better care for menopausal women. Some, though not many, physicians began to engage in the research from which concrete answers might come. Organizations such as the North American Menopause Society and the National Osteoporosis Foundation, to name just two, were formed to increase interest in menopausal women and their concerns. The government got involved and launched the Women's Health Initiative.

Little by little, more is being understood about how women age. In 1996, when the first crush of baby boomers became fifty, the momentum picked up, and the demand for research and information escalated. But scientific solutions are not the sole answer to improving postmenopausal women's lives. Women must pitch in to eradicate forever the perception of postmenopausal women as being over the hill. The challenge to women everywhere is to begin today to appreciate the value of their experiences, their wisdom, and their outer and inner beauty.

PART FOUR

Making the Decision

13

So . . . Should I Take Estrogen?

S FAR as I am concerned the naysayers are doing as much damage as the promoters of estrogen. If I were you I would trust only myself to make the decision. It pays for each of us to get in touch with and listen carefully first and foremost to ourselves. If your inner self is crying out "This is not me. I want to be me again," you must heed the message and try to understand what the menopausal transition has changed in you. Then you must begin to form your decision about how to help yourself.

Of course, in order to do that you need to do some research. You cannot just depend on a health care professional to take you by the hand and lead you down the path to good health and a long life. The medical profession has polarized itself, with physicians on either end of the spectrum giving women advice from where a particular physician is standing at a particular time. There is no question that you do need to work with your physician to get information and medical care, but you also need to search out information by yourself. If you are having symptoms that you know seem like menopause and feel like menopause, they probably are perimenopausal symptoms. Yet physician after physician will give women the pat line "You are much too young for menopause." But with eight out of a hundred women going through early menopause, that is, menopause before the age of forty, how can they be sure?

They can't. So ask for a follicle-stimulating hormone (FSH) blood test. If you must, demand one. But what if that test doesn't show an elevation in the FSH? If you know something strange is going on, I suggest that you ask for another FSH test to be performed at another time of the month. If the two tests disagree, perhaps a third is indicated. The point of this is that you may find yourself in the position of demanding your diagnosis. I'm convinced that no one knows exactly what is going on inside of you but you.

With appropriate blood testing and analyses of your symptoms, you can discover your stage in the menopause transition. Then the number one question returns to haunt you: "Should I take estrogen?" That answer depends on so many factors: your personal medical history, your family medical history, your symptoms, and, ultimately, your choice. This is the time when you have to be in complete charge of your decision. You have to weigh the risk-to-benefit factors and try to balance them. Assistance would be nice at this point, and this is when you need to make sure that you have a good physician-partner, one who wants to work with you so that you can comfortably and safely arrive at your own decision. That partner should respect your decision and be willing to work with it while also providing you with new scientific information as it becomes available, so that you are always aware of the latest information that might benefit you. I know that with the advent of managed care that task is more difficult than ever, but you *can* find that relationship, and once you have succeeded, it is more than worth it.

134 How do I find my physician-partner?

The truth is, we have to exert some effort. If you can connect with a women's health center, and they are cropping up around the country, you might be able to get all the help you need within a multidisciplinary approach. A survey conducted by the Jacobs Institute for Women's Health in Washington, D.C., found that by 1993 there were some 3,600 such centers in the United States and that the number was growing by 20 percent per year. Often these centers are devoted to primary care and offer a full range of services.

From the surveys I did with women from 1991 to this writing, I learned, not surprisingly, that the two top categories of specialties involved in midlife women's health were gynecologists and general family practitioners or internists. Although many women were comfortable with their physician, an equal number were not. Some women had no idea how to prepare themselves for an office visit so they could derive the most benefit from it; others were concerned about how to change physicians.

In February 1998 I was invited to help launch the new Women's Health Center, created by the Franciscan Health System, in Tacoma, Washington. The center, offering a breadth of services under one roof, was and is dedicated "to helping women understand and successfully manage the medical challenges they face in life." In order to do that, the center has assembled a full range of services including conventional, complementary, and alternative medicine; nonsurgical diagnoses and treatments; a weight-training center; mammography, ultrasound, and bone density testing; counseling, an educational resource center, and a toll-free twenty-four-hour health resource line, which can provide everything from referrals to prescriptions, to over-the-counter drug information. The center's services range from conventional techniques, to acupuncture and biofeedback, to massage and physical therapy, and then some. What a wonderful facility to have in one's own hometown!

There may be more services than you are aware of near where you live. I suggest calling the Medical Society in your area and hospitals near you to see if you can find a center dedicated to your midlife health and wellness, or a physician practice that can refer you to support therapies and groups that can help. I know that a letter to the North American Menopause Society (see appendix D) will bring you the names of centers or physicians in your area who care for women through the menopause transition and beyond.

135 What should I expect from my physician?

You should be able to tell your physician that you are seeking a partner in good health. She or he should agree to a collaborative effort. You should expect someone who will give you the proper workup and who will discuss menopause and HRT or ERT, or the other new drugs like Evista, whichever is appropriate, with you when you have questions, not just hand you a prescription. The physician should explain both the risks and the benefits of each prescription drug.

The tests you are given or that are ordered for you during your annual visit to your primary care physician or gynecologist should include blood pressure, blood cholesterol, blood sugar, bone density, breast exam, pelvic exam, Pap test, and mammogram. Bone density testing is not needed repeatedly if your test results demonstrate no bone loss and you are taking estrogen or Evista.

136 What services are usually available in a multidisciplinary women's center?

A good women's center should have many kinds of specialists who could at some time be involved in your care. The ideal would be that you had not only one-stop shopping, but first-rate one-stop shopping. The center should have on call primary care physicians or specialists in internal medicine, gynecologists, endocrinologists, gastroenterologists, dermatologists, urologists, psychotherapists, physical therapists, and specialists in nutrition and exercise. You should be able to obtain all your tests and whatever other procedures are required for you. Many centers, like the new one in Tacoma, also incorporate some of the alternative treatments. The center's hours should be convenient to women's schedules, including some early morning or evening hours and, perhaps, some time slots on the weekends. A center such as this should always have staff on-call to assist you should an emergency arise.

137 What kind of educational materials should I seek?

You need to read more than one book or one article about issues that are important to you. Keep a file with the information you have gathered and refer to it periodically. You want to learn all you can about mammography, how often it should be done and how fast you should get the results. You should become familiar with bone density testing and learn what kind of test you are being offered and what the possibilities for error are, as well as how frequently the test should be repeated. You need to know everything you can about estrogen and the other hormones like progesterone, testosterone, and those secreted by the thyroid gland, which some women replace after menopause. You want to be fully informed about selective estrogen receptor modulators (SERMs) like Evista. You want to know what the results of your Pap test mean and about any false positives or negatives that can show up on the test. The best thing you can do is read divergent points of view on these and other health care topics and discuss them with your physician-partner. Your physician should always be willing to substantiate why he or she is suggesting a specific course of action for you.

What I'm asking you to do is to bring something to the party. By that I mean before you go into your physician's office, spend some time getting ready. First list your questions, and then any problems you might be having. Read up on the subjects you will be broaching during the appointment. In that way you can get the best medical advice in the least amount of time.

138 Can I find health information services on the Internet?

There is a wealth of health information on the Internet. The computer network can be your first source when you want to know more about certain physicians in your area, when you want details concerning a particular disease or medical condition, to check drug interactions, and to learn of suggested treatments and modalities of care for certain illnesses. The problem is that the Internet's information is not always reliable.

The World Wide Web pages are particularly interesting and a good place to begin your search for health information. There are sites on the Web devoted to providing health information in general as well as those devoted to just about every disease. There are pages set up by many medical organizations, women's health groups, hospitals, and medical schools at universities; I have even set up an informational web page (see chapter 15).

139 What are some reliable web sites when it comes to women's midlife health?

Here are a few quality web sites:
National Institutes of Health (*http://www.nih.gov*)
U.S. Food and Drug Administration (FDA) (*http://www.fda.gov*)
American Cancer Society (http://www.cancer.org)
American Heart Association (*http://www.amhrt.org*)
U.S. Government (*www.healthfinder.gov*)
America Online has set up a very reliable site especially for women who would like to discuss menopause. It's called Power Surge. It was created and is hosted by a bright, caring woman named Alice Stamm, who twice a week hosts a chat room and invites experts in the field of women's health as guests to answer questions for her large following of "surgettes." I've been a guest on Power Surge many times and enjoy the opportunity to share information. The keyword is *powersurge@thrive.com*. You can also visit Alice's web site at www.dearest.com. There's much to learn from Alice, her guests, and the women who fill her chat room.

140 What do I do if instead of being told I'm perimenopausal, I'm told I need a hysterectomy?

First find out why you "need a hysterectomy." Then get a second opinion. This double check should not offend your surgeon, who may be willing to assist you in locating another surgeon who will review your case. Or you may feel more secure in selecting your own. Many insurance companies require a second opinion anyway, so don't be concerned about getting one. It is in your best interest.

It is also important that you be an educated consumer. You need to know that if your uterus and both your ovaries are removed, surgical menopause will result. In medical terms that is called a hysterectomy with a bilateral oophorectomy. If you jump back to chapter 1 and reread the mechanics of menopause, you will note that it begins when the ovaries have run out of eggs and the production of the female sex hormones, estrogen and progesterone, has diminished greatly or ceased altogether. When both ovaries are removed and the hormones are suddenly gone, you will be quickly thrust into menopause. Menopausal symptoms can begin suddenly and intensely. You have a lot to consider before you submit to the surgery, including whether you can be given estrogen, and perhaps a touch of testosterone, immediately, which should provide you with a fairly seamless transition into menopause. Ask lots of questions and take your time. Check out the Internet, too. There are a number of good books about hysterectomy that you may wish to read. Dr. Vicki Hufnagel's *No More Hysterectomies* is one choice.

I am wary of hysterectomies, because more than 600,000 such surgical procedures have, in the recent past, been performed in the United States each year, and the report that perhaps two-thirds of them were unnecessary is unsettling. The median age of the woman undergoing the procedure is forty and a half. That's long before natural menopause should occur, and deprives the body of hormones way too soon. Hysterectomy remains the most frequently performed surgical procedure on women in the United States, and because premature aging quickly begins afterward, caution should be your watchword. Take your time. The need for an emergency hysterectomy is rare.

The Centers for Disease Control (CDC) reports that uterine fibroids is the most common reason for performing a hysterectomy, followed by endometriosis, prolapse, cancer, and endometrial hyperplasia. These may be good reasons, but still, consider the surgery carefully. There can be some long-term, long-lasting effects of hysterectomy with bilateral oophorectomy. Many women, between one third and one half, suffer from some form of minor depression following the procedure. Some women complain that their libido disappeared, never to return, taking with it the quality of their orgasms; that their hot flashes and night sweats are intolerable; and that they are fighting a losing battle with weight gain.

There are a number of less dramatic ways to solve some of the problems that heretofore have indicated hysterectomy. Now there are procedures such as myomectomy, which involves removing fibroids by going through either the cervix or the abdomen into the uterus while leaving the uterus intact; dilatation and curettage (D&C), which scrapes away the lining of the uterus; and endometrial ablation, which uses electrical cautery to destroy the lining of the uterus. The newest nonsurgical procedure takes thirty minutes and uses a balloon to deliver heat to the lining of the uterus, destroying the lining and thus reducing bleeding. More than a third of hysterectomies are performed each year because of menorrhagia, or excessive menstrual bleeding. Discuss the other options with your surgeon. Depending on the reason for your procedure, you may be able to consider one of them. Hysterectomy should be the last resort. It is major surgery!

141 How can I get my doctor to consider my concerns and questions seriously?

Take your self seriously. Always present yourself as confident and the issues that you wish to discuss as important. Too frequently, we women don't want to appear to be complainers, so we lightly toss off questions and comments in our effort to disguise our real concerns. That's a big mistake. In our effort to appear lighthearted we lose sight of the seriousness of our office visit. Another mistake women frequently make, and I have been guilty of this, as well, is that when the white-coated physician enters the room and pleasantly says, "How are you?" we say "Fine." That is the wrong answer, because from then on we have to back-pedal to get to the point of our visit. What we should say to get the visit off to a productive start is "I am here because . . . ," and launch right into our list of concerns, pleasantly but directly. There is no time for chitchat here, just the business of getting good medical care. If the physician is a friend or family member, save chat time for the end of the visit, if the doctor has time. Do not risk wasting your valuable consultation time on small talk. That's a rule that I follow, and I have learned well how to make the most of the very few minutes that doctors have for each patient.

I have also found a fairly successful way to get around the issue of postexamination consultation, which formerly was held between me in my flimsy paper dress and my fully clothed, confidant physician. What I have done on occasion, when a longer discussion is required at the end of my visit, is suggest the following, always pleasantly: "Doctor, since I'm uncomfortable discussing something so important in this situation, can we level the playing field? Either you wait until I get dressed and can meet you in your office, or you get undressed and we talk here." If your doctor has a decent sense of humor, you'll meet in the office a few minutes later. If not, you will still have made your point—and it is an important one.

142 How can I get my life's partner involved in my pursuit of good health and a good doctor to steer me through my menopausal years?

Men really have a tough time understanding women's menopausal symptoms. There is nothing in the male physiology that can compare with women's loss of certain hormones. So I suggest you make your mate your confidant, but share the experience of menopause with him only in small bites. It would be unfair and practically impossible to expect a mate to understand all of women's physiology and psychology in one sitting.

I always suggest that you start by asking your partner to read a paragraph or two in a menopause book that you think is pertinent to what you wish to discuss, and use that as a spring-board to your dialogue. Or circle a section in a newspaper or magazine article and use that to open a particular discussion.

My experience has shown that most men really do try to understand and work with their spouses on some of the issues that surround the menopause transition. I also now see many more men accompanying their wives at my lectures, trying to learn and trying to help. So don't cut your partner out, but do cut him some slack in terms of how much he can or wants to absorb at one time.

Your partner can be of inestimable assistance in your search for your physician-partner, so keep him in the loop. Let him accompany you to your first consultation with the doctor if you are having a particularly rough time handling your symptoms. I know for me it is very comforting to know that my husband is participating with me in my search for continued good health.

143 I'm tired all the time and my partner thinks I'm trying to avoid him. Will estrogen help?

Estrogen does have a mental tonic effect on some women. A touch of testosterone can also lift fatigue. But if you're feeling exhausted lately, like you're driving on empty or your get-up-and-go simply got up and went, have your thyroid checked. The answer to your problem may be just under your Adam's apple. There lies your thyroid gland, the little accelerator to your gas pedal. The thyroid controls the tempo of all our body's processes, for example, heartbeat, thought, and digestion. When the thyroid changes the amount of hormone it secretes, we suffer. It can go too fast, causing hyperthyroidism; or too slow, causing hypothyroidism. In either case, it's a problem and one out of five women at some point develops an out-of-sync thyroid and often does not realize it. So if you have been feeling tired for a long time, see your physician and have your thyroid checked. There's an inexpensive, simple blood test called TSH, or thyroid stimulating hormone assay, that can show whether your thyroid is functioning in a normal range. An underactive thyroid, hypothyroidism, affects 20 to 25 percent of women over the age of sixty.

144 What are the symptoms of hypothyroidism?

Fatigue, weight gain, chills, constipation, poor concentration, muscle cramping, dry skin, thinning hair, brittle nails, extreme sensitivity to cold, and even a problem with swallowing all can indicate a thyroid that's slowing down. Since some of these symptoms may also be common to aging, it's easy for you and your physician to pass them off. Don't! An underactive thyroid can cause all kinds of problems, including a hike in cholesterol levels, which can increase your risk of heart disease. It might be a good idea for women to get a baseline thyroid test (a TSH) as early as age thirty-five or forty, since most people with thyroid problems are unaware that they have them. Since it's easy to bring a sluggish thyroid up to par with a synthetic thyroid hormone tablet taken once each day, why not check it out if you are feeling as if your old peppy self has changed into a tired couch potato.

It is important to communicate how you feel. Your spouse can really help if you take him into your confidence. A close friend can help as well. Often just the presence of your significant other in the physician's office can help get to the heart of the matter quickly, and two heads are better than one when you are trying to remember and rethink the discussion that was held and the medical decisions that were made. Your physician will help, too, but only if he or she is aware of how you feel. So, speak up!

145 How do I avoid scare tactics?

Weigh carefully all the facts before you decide upon a course of action. This is valuable advice concerning all things in life, but nothing is more precious than your health. So often we women are fearful of being labeled "hypersensitive," "neurotic," "panic-stricken," "hysterical," "suspicious," or of being called a nervous Nellie, or worse yet, a hypochondriac, that we back off from getting all the information we need and the help we may need in order to make good health care decisions. Do not accept any of these labels, do not doubt yourself, and do not permit your symptoms to be tossed off as being "all in your head."

Here's just one example of what becoming frightened can do to us. One of my readers read the report of a study stating that estrogen causes breast cancer. She stopped taking estrogen cold turkey. Big mistake! Two weeks later another study refuted the earlier one. She called me in tears. "What should I do now?" she said. I told her to call her doctor and discuss the situation. Further, I suggested that she never react to any major news pertaining to her health without discussing it with her health care provider. That's a good suggestion for all of us.

14

How Do I Stay on Track?

B ECOME your own best friend. Weigh carefully all the facts before you decide a course of action. This is valuable advice concerning all things in life, but nothing is more precious than your health. Make sure you adopt lifestyles that will serve you well. Find a physician-partner with whom you are comfortable. Prepare for your office visit by having your questions and your symptoms clearly outlined, in your mind or on a piece of paper. Read all you can about midlife women's health. Stay abreast of the latest medical breakthroughs.

Don't react to medical news without checking it out with your physician. Check with your physician before you discontinue any prescription medication, like estrogen, and learn how to do it properly.

The last chapter of a book such as this is usually a wrap-up. By necessity it contains information that women are concerned about that didn't fit into earlier chapters. So I am going to bounce around a bit to get the last of the 150 most frequently asked questions answered. These last few questions deal with some of the concerns that women continue to have as they attempt to reach their decisions concerning hormone replacement therapy or nonhormonal therapy and how to stay on track.

146 **I keep forgetting to take my estrogen pills and I'm scared to death about doubling up on them. What should I do?**

Devise a system that works for you. Like many other women, you probably subconsciously don't want to have to depend on long-term medication. That's understandable. Yet you do yourself harm if you upset the hormonal balance that your HRT or ERT is establishing. Skipped pills may result in an onrush of menopause symptoms, usually starting with hot flashes, and might cause break-through bleeding, which is a cause for concern. Create a system for taking your daily oral medications: combine it with another activity that you perform almost by rote, such as brushing your teeth. Tie a ribbon on your toothbrush to jolt your pill-taking memory. Or put a sign on the refrigerator or coffee maker if the kitchen is your first stop in the morning. Another avenue you may wish to explore is to try either Prempro or Premphase, which are the newer two-pills-in-one, or the new CombiPatch, if you are on HRT. Or how about considering one of the patches that last a week, like Climara or Fempatch, or the new Estring that stays in place for about three months? These methods require a lot less daily vigilance on your part. Of course, if forgetfulness is your problem, you'll have to devise a tracking system for these forms of estrogen as well. Think every Monday for the once-a-week patch, or mark your calendar for the first of each third month for the ring. You get the idea.

147 **My physician keeps steering me away from micronized progesterone and telling me to "stick with a winner." I'm miserable on progestin and scared to insist on the change. Why is getting micronized progesterone prescribed such a challenge?**

It's unbelievable that this type of problem still exists almost a decade after menopause and women's health issues have moved to the front burner! But it does exist, and the reason is undoubtedly because there is not yet an oral micronized progesterone product approved by the FDA for use in HRT. Your physician is being cautious because of that, and more important, because there have not been extensive controlled scientific studies on micronized progesterone, so the amount appropriate for protecting the endometrium has not been finally established. There is little doubt that for many women, the oral micronized progesterone is far superior to synthetic progestin, primarily in relieving the menopause blues. You can obtain this product with your physician's prescription from one of the many compounding pharmacies. A call to the National Association of Compounding Pharmacists (1-800-687-7694) will give you the name of one close to you. Then call the pharmacy and ask them to send information concerning this product to both you and your physician. Let your doctor know it is coming. Once you've both learned more about it, perhaps your doctor will order it for you. As mentioned earlier Solvay Pharmaceuticals has an application under review by the FDA and will probably be offering oral micronized progesterone.

148 I am taking estrogen, but I am still afraid I will lose my husband because I have lost my sexual appetite. What can I do?

That is a real fear, expressed by many women. Their libido is gone, and even though they participate in sexual intercourse they fear that their husband of many years is aware of their lack of interest. It is excruciatingly painful to be caught up in that kind of fear, because every flirtatious woman at a party, every secretary at his office, and every model on television or in newspaper or magazine ads appears to be a threat. This is the time to take your problem to your physician and discuss what you can do to reawaken your sexual desire. Often a little testosterone added to your hormone cocktail is all that you need to fix this problem. Also, instead of hiding it from your partner, perhaps enlisting his help would be more advantageous and you would feel better about it. Share not only your current situation, but also material in this book and others that show how common the problem is, and talk about the fact that it is not about less love for him, it's about fewer hormones in you. Let him know you will seek medical help to correct the problem. In most relationships, this kind of honesty works. Today, because this problem is so common, there are more ways to take testosterone than ever before. Besides the pills, injections, and pellets mentioned earlier, there is also a 2 percent testosterone cream that can be applied to the female genitalia with amazingly good results.

149 All of a sudden my hair is limp and is thinning. Will some specific kind of estrogen help?

Alas, this is also a common problem. The good news is that there is help. My dermatologist, Dr. Wilma Bergfeld, director of dermapathology at the Cleveland Clinic and a former president of the American Dermatological Association, offers her patients an estrogen solution that is topically applied to the scalp wherever hair is thinning. I am happy to tell you that it works!

The follicle for each hair on our heads is located deep in our dermis, or skin. The hair follicle stays in place because it is supported by collagen-rich tissue, which is maintained by estrogen. As we age and lose estrogen, the amount of collagen we make tends to diminish, which can make our skin thinner and dryer. While this is going on, the fat and muscle under the skin can also shrink. When these important tissues no longer do a first-rate job, hair loss can result. Do not just suffer in silence. Do discuss this with a dermatologist, who, I am sure, will be able to help.

Since we've raised the issue of collagen and skin, let's spend a moment discussing the impact of menopause on our smooth and rosy, glowing skin. Collagen is a necessary protein in the skin. Skin cells, like bones in our younger years, continue to replenish themselves. As we age, that process slows, the layer of fat cells under the skin shrinks somewhat, and our skin loses some of its youthful elasticity and begins to wrinkle. You should be able to prevent much of the change in your skin. First of all, the sun is your skin's worst enemy. Stay out of it. It dries your skin, causing wrinkles and creases, and creates those brown spots of aging. Smoking is also tough on your skin and is often responsible for vertical wrinkles around the mouth. So what can you do? Don't smoke. Keep your skin moist. Wear sunscreen every single day. Drink lots of water, which helps to plump up the skin, and consider estrogen. Estrogen helps enormously to keep the skin smooth, supple, and young looking.

150 How can I learn to love this time of life?

How can you not love this time of life? You are free. It's a time to celebrate. If they have not already disappeared, menstrual periods and cramps will soon be a distant memory along with fear of an unwanted pregnancy. Many women around the time of menopause know exactly who they are for the first time in their lives. Never before has medical science provided us with such an exciting future, informing us that a woman who is healthy at fifty may well live into her eighties, or that a woman healthy at sixty may live into her nineties or even longer. Never before has there been so much research on women's health. Never before has the subject of menopause been so out in the open, and information so readily available. Never before have we had so many choices to counteract menopause's physical and psychological changes.

There is a new respect for the woman at midlife. She is accomplished, and she is still accomplishing. The late actress Helen Hayes is reported to have said, "Rest is rust." I believe that, and so do many, many enlightened postmenopausal women. In earlier books I would list in a paragraph or two the names of women past fifty that you would readily recognize whose careers have soared. Today there are so many age fifty-plus women in the public eye that a whole book could be devoted to listing them. One thing I know for sure. We are not "invisible," as feminist Germaine Greer once proclaimed. Menopause does not mean we are at the end of anything. In fact, we are just beginning what can and should be the most wonderful time of our lives.

Estrogen Decision Self-Evaluation "Test"

I have the following menopause symptoms. They alter the quality of my life (rank symptoms from 1 to 10, with 1 being barely bothersome and 10 indicating that they are debilitating). Then assign every symptom that achieves a 6 or higher number 10 points. Assign 5 points to every symptom that ranks between 1 and 5.

Short-term symptoms

_____ hot flashes
_____ night sweats
_____ vaginal dryness
_____ insomnia
_____ heart palpitations
_____ anxiety
_____ mood swings
_____ fatigue
_____ lack of libido
_____ joint pain
_____ Other (list) _____
                       _____
                       _____

Analyze your score as follows:

10–20	No big problem.
20–40	I guess I can live with them.
40–60	This is not fun.
60–80	I need help. The quality of my life is diminished.
80–100 or more	My symptoms are making me non-functional.

Long-term prevention

Check the risk factors that apply to you and give each check 4 points. I have a family history of

_____ breast cancer
_____ colon/rectal cancer
_____ other cancers
_____ heart disease
_____ osteoporosis
_____ Alzheimer's disease
_____ osteoarthritis

I have a personal history of

_____ breast cancer
_____ other cancers
_____ endometriosis
_____ heart disease
_____ osteoporosis
_____ osteoarthritis
_____ gallbladder disease
_____ liver disease
_____ phlebitis or other circulatory disease
_____ I experienced an early menopause (before age forty).
_____ I am Caucasian or Asian.
_____ I am small boned and thin.
_____ I am sedentary.
_____ I have had a lifelong calcium deficiency.
_____ I take medications that contribute to loss of bone mineral density.
_____ I smoke.
_____ I am a heavy drinker.

Analyze your score as follows:

10–20 points	I can forgo conventional HRT or ERT.
20–40 points	I could go either way.
40–60 points	Maybe I should consider estrogen.
60–80 points	Estrogen replacement therapy is looking good.
80–100 points	I should take estrogen.

15

Let's Stay in Touch!

N ALL of my books, I offer open lines of communication between my readers and me. How else can one truly be a
women's health advocate? Over the years, I have been in touch
with thousands of women, some only once, others whenever
a new question arises for them. Some women write to share their
experiences; others seek advice or help. I relish this two-way communication. First, I know on a daily basis that somewhere I am
helping someone. Second, readers' letters keep me abreast of
what's going on in the wide world of women and what new questions women have about their midlife health and wellness. From
this interactive relationship, I know we can learn more about how
to create for ourselves that first-rate second half of adult life we
all seek.

Your medical needs must be provided for by a medical doctor, and I hope I have encouraged you sufficiently to search for
and acquire the patient-physician partnership that will benefit
your health and assure you good medical care. You and I can
have a different kind of sharing, that which provides each of us
with important information so that we can remain educated and
empowered to get the best care possible as well as to be knowledgeable about the lifestyles that have worked for others and may
work for us. We all want to know about medical and nonmedical
self-help methods. We also want to be fully informed about hormonal and nonhormonal treatments from which we can choose.

My address is below. I look forward to hearing from you. I am happy to receive your comments, questions, and suggestions, which enable me to write books and magazine articles that respond appropriately to women's current needs. I can't promise to answer each of your letters personally, but I can promise you that your area of concern will be included in the basketful of ideas for my next book or for my column, "Woman to Woman," in *Your Health* magazine (see appendix B).

I am sorry that I cannot provide you with referrals to menopause specialists in your area, but a quick look in Appendix D will let you know of organizations that can. If there is a menopause or an osteoporosis society in your country, that is a good place to start. For example, The North American Menopause Society, which is listed, can help you with referrals in the United States, Canada, and, perhaps, even elsewhere. These organizations prefer that you write to them rather than call.

I hope you will want to share your thoughts and ideas. Together we can continue to help other women, especially those baby boomers who are joining us in this new and wonderful stage of life.

You can write to me at the following address:
Ruth S. Jacobowitz
10951 Sorrento Valley Road, Suite 1-D
San Diego, CA 92121
E-mail: ruthsj@san.rr.com
You can also check out my web site at
www.ruthjacobowitz.com.

An Osteoporosis-Prevention Calcium Counter*

This calcium counter is for women and men of all ages, to show how easy it is to find calcium if you know where to look. Science has shown us that we can continue to build bone until the age of thirty to thirty-five. Then we begin to lose bone at the rate of about 1 percent per year. For women in the seven to ten years following menopause, bone loss can accelerate from 1 percent per year to 3 percent per year or more.

A calcium-rich diet is vital to building and maintaining bone. The recommended daily allowance for calcium for women is as follows:

1,000 milligrams per day from puberty to menopause

1,200 milligrams per day if you are pregnant or breast feeding

1,500 milligrams per day if you are postmenopausal and not taking estrogen

1,500 milligrams after age sixty-five whether you take estrogen or not

Those numbers seem to indicate that it is necessary to eat an abundance of dairy products known to be calcium-rich foods. That is not so if you know which other calcium-rich foods to choose. This calcium counter has been prepared to help you find foods that have at least 50

*Prepared by Ruth S. Jacobowitz with the assistance of Deanne Siegal, M.S., R.D. Values for this counter were obtained from Bowes and Church's "Food Values of Portions Commonly Used," 15th edition; product labels; and the fast-food industry.

milligrams of calcium per serving. To assist you further in pursuing healthful eating, it also includes the total fat and calorie count of each serving.

	Serving	Calcium (mg)	Calories	Fat (g)
BREADS, BREAD PRODUCTS, AND FLOURS				
barley, pearled, pot/scotch	1 cup	68	696	2.2
Bisquick baking and pancake mix	1/2 cup	80	240	8.0
bran muffin, homemade	1 small	54	112	5.1
bread, wheat, Home Pride, Light	2 slices	120	70	1.0
bread, wheat/nine-grain, Wonder Light	2 slices	160	80	<1.0
bread, wheat, Home Pride	2 slices	80	140	2.0
bread, white, Wonder	2 slices	80	140	2.0
bun, hamburger/hot dog	1 bun	54	114	2.1
carob flour	1 cup	493	452	2.0
cornbread, from mix	1 piece	133	178	5.8
corn flour, masa harina, Quaker	1/3 cup	77	137	1.5
corn meal, enriched, self-rising	1/6 cup	109	99	0.9
corn meal mix, Aunt Jemima	1/6 cup	60	99	0.7
corn muffin, from mix	1 small	96	130	4.2
English muffin, plain	1	92	135	1.1
French toast, frozen, Aunt Jemima	2 slices	94	168	3.9
hoagie bun	1 large roll, 5.9 oz.	252	470	8.4
pancakes, buttermilk, from mix, Hungry Jack	3 pancakes	154	180	1.0
pancakes, frozen, Aunt Jemima	3 pancakes	66	246	3.7

	Serving	Calcium (mg)	Calories	Fat (g)
BREADS, BREAD PRODUCTS, AND FLOURS, *continued*				
pancakes, frozen batter, Aunt Jemima	3 pancakes	68	210	1.6
pancakes, frozen prepared, Aunt Jemima Lite	3 pancakes	250	140	2.0
pancake/waffle mix, buckwheat, Aunt Jemima	1/4 cup dry	150	107	0.8
pancake/waffle mix, buttermilk, Aunt Jemima	1/3 cup dry	230	175	0.7
pita bread	1.75 oz.	120	120	<1.0
rice bran, Ener-G foods	3.5 oz.	355	438	21.7
rye flour, dark	1 cup	69	419	3.3
soybean flour, defatted	1 cup	241	327	1.2
soybean flour, full fat	1 cup	175	368	17.6
soy meal, defatted	1 cup	297	411	2.9
spoonbread w/white ground corn meal	1 cup	230	468	27.4
waffles, frozen prepared, Aunt Jemima Lite	1 waffle	100	80	1.0
wheat flour, all purpose, enriched, Pillsbury's Best	1 cup	238	401	0.9
CEREALS, COOKED OR TO BE COOKED				
Maypo, cooked	3/4 cup	94	128	1.8
oatmeal, Quaker instant plain	1 packet	150	100	2.0
oatmeal, Quaker instant w/ fruit flavor	1 packet	150	150[a]	2.0
oatmeal, Quaker instant w/ maple and brown sugar	1 packet	200	140	2.0

[a] *Average for fruit flavors*

CEREALS, READY TO EAT				
Basic Four, General Mills	3/4 cup	200	130	2.0
Just Right, Kellogg's crunchy nugget	2/3 cup	200	110	1.0

	Serving	Calcium (mg)	Calories	Fat (g)
CEREALS, READY TO EAT, *continued*				
Just Right, Kellogg's fruit and nut	3/4 cup	200	140	1.0
Life cereals, Quaker	2/3 cup	60	110	1.8
Muesli, Alpen	1/2 cup	80	220	3.0
Total, General Mills	1 cup	200	110	0.6
Total Raisin Bran, General Mills	1 cup	200	140	1.0
CHEESE AND CHEESE PRODUCTS				
Alpine Lace Free 'N Lean slices	1 oz.	200	40	0.0
Alpine Lace Swiss	1 oz.	250	90	6.0
American, processed	1 oz.	124	106	8.9
blue	1 oz.	150	100	8.2
Borden Fat-Free slices	1 oz.	200	40	0.0
Borden Lite Line slices	2/3 oz.	150	25	0.0
brick	1 oz.	191	105	8.4
Brie	1 oz.	52	95	7.9
Camembert	1 oz.	110	85	6.9
caraway-seeded	1 oz.	191	107	8.3
cheddar	1 oz.	204	114	9.4
cheese fondue, homemade	1/4 cup	203	170	11.2
cheese nuggets, cheddar, frozen, Banquet	3 oz.	328	414	30.0
cheese nuggets, mozzarella, frozen, Banquet	3 oz.	355	288	16.0
cheese sauce, canned, Campbell's	2 oz.	63	60	4.1
cheese sauce, from dry mix	1/2 cup	285	158	8.5
Cheez Whiz, Kraft	1 oz.	100	80	6.0
Cheshire	1 oz.	182	110	8.7
Colby	1 oz.	194	112	9.1
cottage cheese, creamed	1/2 cup	68	117	5.1

	Serving	Calcium (mg)	Calories	Fat (g)
CHEESE AND CHEESE PRODUCTS, *continued*				
cottage cheese, 1% fat	1/2 cup	68	80	1.0
cottage cheese, 2% fat	1/2 cup	75	100	2.2
Edam	1 oz.	207	101	7.9
feta	1 oz.	140	75	6.0
fontina	1 oz.	156	110	8.8
Formagg slices	3/4 oz.	250	70	5.0
gjetost	1 oz.	113	132	8.4
Gouda	1 oz.	198	191	7.8
Gruyère	1 oz.	287	117	9.2
havarti	1 oz.	176	121	10.0
Healthy Choice American	1 oz.	200	40	0.0
Healthy Choice Mozzarella	1 oz.	250	40	0.0
Kraft Fat-Free slices	1 oz.	200	45	0.0
Kraft Health Favorites slices	2/3 oz.	200	45	2.0
Kraft Light Naturals	1 oz.	250	80	5.0
Kraft Light 'N Lively	1 oz.	200	70	4.0
Laughing Cow	1 wedge	100	70	6.0
Laughing Cow, light	1 wedge	150	50	3.0
Limburger	1 oz.	141	93	7.7
Monterey Jack	1 oz.	212	106	8.6
mozzarella	1 oz.	147	80	6.1
mozzarella, part-skim	1 oz.	183	72	4.9
Muenster	1 oz.	203	104	8.5
Parmesan, grated	1 T	69	23	1.5
Parmesan, hard	1 oz.	336	111	7.3
Port du Salut	1 oz.	184	100	8.0
provolone	1 oz.	214	100	7.6
ricotta, light	4 oz.	160	80	4.0
ricotta, part-skim	4 oz.	337	171	9.8
ricotta, whole milk	4 oz.	257	216	16.1
Romano	1 oz.	302	110	7.6
Roquefort, sheep's milk	1 oz.	188	105	8.7

	Serving	Calcium (mg)	Calories	Fat (g)
Shedd's Country Crock cheddar spread	1 oz.	200	70	4.0
Swiss	1 oz.	272	107	7.8
Swiss, processed	1 oz.	219	95	7.1
Tilsit, whole milk	1 oz.	198	96	7.4
Velveeta, Kraft	1 oz.	150	80	6.0
Velveeta light, Kraft	1 oz.	100	70	4.0
Weight Watchers, slices	4/5 oz.	150	50	2.0
DESSERTS *Cakes*				
Boston cream pie[a]	1/8 cake	69	311	9.7
double fudge cake, frozen, Weight Watchers	2.75 oz.	60	180	4.0
Duncan Hines cake mix[b]	1/12 cake	60	250	10.0
Duncan Hines DeLights cake mix[b]	1/12 cake	60	180	5.0
lemon cake mix, Betty Crocker	1/12 cake	80	260	11.0
Cookies				
oatmeal apple, Grandma's	2 cookies	60	330	12.0
Custard				
baked homemade	1 cup	297	305	14.6
Frozen desserts				
caramel fudge a la mode, Weight Watchers	1	80	180	3.0
caramel nut bar, Weight Watchers	2 oz.	80	120	7.0
Fudgsicle	1.75 oz.	60	70	1.0
Fudgsicle, sugar-free	1.75 oz.	60	35	1.0
frozen dessert, Baskin-Robbins, Fat-Free[b]	4 oz.	100	100	0.0

	Serving	Calcium (mg)	Calories	Fat (g)
DESSERTS, *continued*				
frozen dessert, Baskin-Robbins Lite[b]	4 oz.	100	130	6.0
frozen dessert, Baskin-Robbins sugar-free[b]	4 oz.	100	80	1.0
frozen dessert, Eskimo Pie, sugar-free	4 oz.	100	130	7.0
frozen dessert, Healthy Choice[b]	4 oz.	100	130	2.0
frozen dessert, Simple Pleasures Light[b]	4 oz.	100	90	1.0
frozen dessert, Weight Watchers[b]	4 oz.	100	80	0.0
frozen yogurt, Ben and Jerry's[b]	3 oz.	100	120	1.0
frozen yogurt, Häagen-Dazs[b]	4 oz.	150	180	4.0
frozen yogurt, Edy's, fat-free[b]	4 oz.	120	90	0.0
frozen yogurt, Ruggles[b]	3 oz.	80	90	2.0
frozen yogurt, TCBY[b]	4 oz.	80	130	3.0
frozen yogurt, TCBY, nonfat[b]	4 oz.	80	110	0.0
frozen yogurt, TCBY, sugar-free[b]	4 oz.	100	80	<1.0
ice cream, Baskin-Robbins[b]	4 oz.	150	240	14.0
ice cream, Breyers[b]	4 oz.	100	160	8.0
ice cream, Häagen-Dazs[b]	4 oz.	100	280	17.0
ice cream bar, Eskimo Pie	3 oz.	60	180	12.0
ice cream bar, Eskimo Pie, sugar-free	2½ oz.	80	140	11.0
ice cream bar, Häagen-Dazs[b]	1 bar	100	370	27.0
ice cream bar, Klondike Lite	2½ oz.	100	110	6.0
ice cream drumstick	1	100	220	10.0
ice cream sandwich	1	73	169	6.2
ice milk, vanilla	4 oz.	85	110	3.0
mousse pop, Weight Watchers	1.75 oz.	60	35	<1.0

	Serving	Calcium (mg)	Calories	Fat (g)
DESSERTS, *continued*				
pudding pops, Jell-O	1.75 oz.	80	70	2.0
sherbet, orange	4 oz.	52	135	1.9
vanilla sandwich bar, Weight Watchers	2.75 oz.	150	160	4.0
yogurt shake, Weight Watchers	7.5 oz.	250	220	1.0
Pastries				
cream puff w/custard filling	1	105	303	18.1
eclair w/custard filling, chocolate icing	1	80	239	13.6
toaster pastry, vitamin-fortified, Merico	1	150	220	7.0
Pies				
banana cream	1/8 pie	67	233	11.9
butterscotch	1/8 pie	86	304	12.5
chocolate cream	1/8 pie	96	301	17.3
chocolate mousse, from mix, Jell-O[c]	1/8 pie	74	249	14.6
coconut cream, from mix, Jello-O[c]	1/8 pie	67	260	16.5
coconut custard	1/8 pie	107	268	14.3
pumpkin	1/8 pie	58	241	12.8
sweet potato	1/8 pie	79	243	12.9
Puddings				
bread, homemade	1/2 cup	149	248	8.2
Hershey's, prepared	1/2 cup	100	180	5.0
Hershey's, fat-free, prepared	1/2 cup	80	100	0.0
Hunts Snack Pack, prepared	1/2 cup	80	160	6.0
Hunts Snack Pack, Light, prepared	1/2 cup	100	100	2.0
Jell-O pudding, from instant mix[c]	1/2 cup	147	165	4.3
Jell-O pudding, sugar-free, from mix[d]	1/2 cup	150	90	2.4

	Serving	Calcium (mg)	Calories	Fat (g)
DESSERTS, *continued*				
rennin dessert, homemade[c]	1/2 cup	142	114	4.5
rice w/raisins, homemade[c]	1/2 cup	130	194	4.1
Slimfast puddings, prepared	1/2 cup	100	100	<1.0
Swiss Miss, prepared	1/2 cup	80	180	6.0
Swiss Miss Light, prepared	1/2 cup	60	100	1.0
tapioca, homemade	1/2 cup	87	110	4.2
Weight Watchers chocolate mousse, from mix[e]	1/2 cup	150	70	3.0
Weight Watchers pudding, from mix[e]	1/2 cup	250	90	0.0

[a] *Layer cake w/custard filling and powdered sugar topping*

[b] *Average for all flavors*

[c] *Made with whole milk*

[d] *Prepared with 2% milk*

[e] *Prepared with skim milk*

CANDY

	Serving	Calcium (mg)	Calories	Fat (g)
caramels, plain/chocolate	4 pieces	55	149	3.9
chocolate chips, milk chocolate	1/4 cup	80	218	11.0
chocolate-covered almonds	1 oz.	57	159	12.2
chocolate kisses	6 pieces	53	154	9.0
chocolate stars	7 pieces	64	145	8.1
golden almond, Hershey	1 oz.	60	161	11.0
Hershey Krackel	1.2 oz.	60	179	9.7
Hershey Whatchamacallit	1.8 oz.	69	270	14.9
Kit Kat	1.5 oz.	65	210	11.0
malted milk balls	14 pieces	63	135	7.0
milk chocolate Chunky	1 oz.	51	120	4.4
milk chocolate, Hershey	1.02 oz.	55	160	9.4

	Serving	Calcium (mg)	Calories	Fat (g)
CANDY, *continued*				
milk chocolate w/almonds, Hershey	1.05 oz.	58	160	9.5
milk chocolate w/fruit and nuts, Cadbury	1 oz.	67	148	8.0
Mr. Goodbar	1.27 oz.	50	198	11.0
raisins w/vanilla yogurt coating	1 oz.	51	134	5.5
Reeses Pieces	1.7 oz.	69	240	10
Rolo	5 pieces	73	139	6.4
EGG DISHES				
omelette, cheese (2 oz.), 3 eggs	1	250	510	37.0
omelette, cheese, from Eggbeaters (Fleishman's)	3.75 oz.	150	110	5.0
omelette sandwich, Weight Watchers[a]	3.84 oz.	175	180	6.0
omelette, vegetable, from Eggbeaters (Fleishman's)	1/2 cup	80	50	0.0
quiche, three cheeses, Pour-A-Quiche	4.3 oz.	289	236	18.7
soufflé, cheese	1 cup	191	207	16.2
soufflé, spinach	1 cup	230	218	18.4

[a] *Average value for all varieties*

ENTREES AND MEALS

Box Mix

	Serving	Calcium (mg)	Calories	Fat (g)
macaroni and cheese dinner, prepared, Kraft	3/4 cup	80	290	13.0
macaroni and cheese deluxe dinner, prepared, Kraft	3/4 cup	123	255	7.5
macaroni and cheese, Slimfast	1 cup	150	230	3.0
NoodleRoni Parmesano/white cheddar shells, prepared, Rice-A-Roni	1/2 cup	80	190	8.0

	Serving	Calcium (mg)	Calories	Fat (g)
NoodleRoni Romanoff, prepared, Rice-A-Roni	1/2 cup	60	220	11.0
pasta and sauce, prepared, Uncle Ben's	1/2 cup	100	170	4.0
pasta shells and cheese, prepared, Velveeta	3/4 cup	186	261	9.8
pizza, cheese, thick crust, Contadina	1/4 pizza	63	295	3.8
pizza, cheese, thin crust, Contadina	1/4 pizza	44	209	3.0
rice w/chicken flavor sauce, Slimfast	8 oz.	150	240	1.0
spaghetti dinner, prepared, Kraft	1 cup	80	310	8.0
Canned Entrees/Side Dishes				
beans, baked, vegetarian	1 cup	80	200	2.0
beans, baked, w/pork	1 cup	120	268	3.9
beans, refried, Chi-Chi's	7.5 oz.	60	250	11.0
chili w/beans	1 cup	119	286	14.0
macaroni and cheese, Franco-American	7.4 oz.	93	168	5.4
ravioli w/meat sauce, Franco-American	7.5 oz.	75	284	10.8
vegetarian chili, mild, Health Valley	5 oz.	80	70	0.0
Frozen Entrees				
angel hair pasta[a]	10 oz.	100	240	5.0
baked cheese ravioli w/ tomato sauce[a]	8½ oz.	200	240	8.0
baked potato w/sour cream[a]	10⅜ oz.	200	230	5.0
beef and bean enchiladas[a]	9¼ oz.	100	240	6.0
beef and vegetables, Banquet	10 oz.	78	300	9.0
beef cannelloni w/tomato sauce[a]	9⅝ oz.	150	200	3.0
beef, chipped and creamed[b]	5.5 oz.	100	230	17.0

	Serving	Calcium (mg)	Calories	Fat (g)

ENTREES AND
MEALS, *continued*

beef ravioli[a]	5 oz.	83	185	5.7
beef Stroganoff w/parsley noodles[b]	9¾ oz.	60	390	20.0
breaded breast of chicken Parmesan[a]	10⅞ oz.	100	200	7.0
broccoli and cheddar baked potato[a]	10⅜ oz.	400	180	9.0
broccoli and cheese baked potato[d]	10.5 oz.	400	270	6.0
cheese blintz	8 oz.	336	432	25.6
cheese cannelloni w/tomato sauce[a]	9⅛ oz.	300	270	8.0
cheese enchiladas[b]	9¾ oz.	600	490	29.0
cheese manicotti[d]	9.25 oz.	350	260	8.0
cheese tortellini[d]	9.0 oz.	200	310	6.0
chicken a la king w/rice[b]	9¼ oz.	80	270	5.0
chicken and vegetables w/ vermicelli[a]	11¾ oz.	80	240	5.0
chicken cordon bleu[e]	7.7 oz.	200	170	5.0
chicken divan[b]	8 oz.	200	220	10.0
chicken enchiladas[a]	9⅞ oz.	150	290	9.0
chicken enchiladas Suez[d]	9.0 oz.	200	230	7.0
chicken fettuccini[a]	9 oz.	150	280	6.0
chicken fettuccini[d]	8.25 oz.	200	280	9.0
chicken fettuccini[f]	8.5 oz.	80	240	4.0
chicken in barbecue sauce w/ rice pilaf[a]	8¾ oz.	60	260	6.0
chicken Miracle[g]	9.2 oz.	60	160	1.0
chicken pie[b]	10 oz.	100	440	27.0
chicken Parmesan dinner	11.5 oz.	100	290	6.0
chicken tenderloins in herb cream sauce[a]	9½ oz.	150	240	5.0
chili con carne w/beans[b]	8¾ oz.	80	280	21.0
creamed chicken[b]	6½ oz.	80	300	17.0

	Serving	Calcium (mg)	Calories	Fat (g)
ENTREES AND MEALS, *continued*				
eggplant Parmesan, Mrs. Paul's	10 oz.	100	240	16.0
escalloped chicken and noodles[b]	10 oz.	100	420	24.0
fettuccini Alfredo[a]	9 oz.	250	280	7.0
fettuccini Alfredo[d]	8.0 oz.	250	230	7.0
fettuccini primavera[a]	10 oz.	300	260	8.0
filet of fish divan[a]	10⅜ oz.	150	210	5.0
filet of fish Florentine[a]	9⅝ oz.	150	220	7.0
French bread pizza[b/c]	6 oz.	200	420	19.0
French bread pizza[a/c]	5⅗ oz.	250	330	10.0
French bread pizza, double cheese[b]	5⅜ oz.	450	420	18.0
French bread pizza, three cheese[a]	5½ oz.	400	330	10.0
French bread pizza, vegetable deluxe[b]	6⁷⁄₁₆ oz.	250	420	20.0
garden lasagna[d]	10¼ oz.	350	260	7.0
garden potato casserole[f]	9.25 oz.	250	180	4.0
grilled chicken sandwich[e]	4 oz.	80	200	5.0
grilled chicken Suez w/ Spanish rice[d]	8.6 oz.	150	220	7.0
herb roasted chicken dinner[f]	11.5 oz.	60	380	7.0
homestyle chicken and noodles[b]	10 oz.	150	290	13.0
homestyle chicken and noodles[d]	9.0 oz.	100	240	7.0
homestyle chicken Parmigiana and pasta alfredo[b]	9⅞ oz.	250	360	15.0
homestyle grilled chicken breast in barbecue sauce[b]	7⅝ oz.	60	210	7.0
homestyle rigatoni and meat sauce[b]	12 oz.	150	400	13.0
homestyle Salisbury steak in gravy and mac & cheese[b]	9⅝ oz.	150	350	17.0

	Serving	Calcium (mg)	Calories	Fat (g)
homestyle spaghetti Parmigiana w/Italian green beans[b]	10¼ oz.	200	240	9.0
homestyle turkey w/ vegetables and pasta[a]	9⅜ oz.	100	230	5.0
homestyle veal Parmigiana and pasta Alfredo[b]	9¼ oz.	250	350	15.0
Jade Garden beef[d]	9.0 oz.	80	150	3.0
lasagna[b]	10 oz.	250	340	12.0
lasagna Florentine[g]	11 oz.	400	220	1.0
lasagna w/meat sauce[a]	10¼ oz.	150	280	6.0
lasagna w/meat sauce[d]	10¼ oz.	400	270	6.0
Lean Pockets, glazed chicken supreme[h]	1 pocket	100	240	7.0
Lean Pockets, turkey, broccoli, and cheese[h]	1 pocket	200	260	9.0
Lean Pockets, sausage and pepperoni pizza deluxe[h]	1 pocket	200	300	11.0
macaroni and beef[d]	9 oz.	80	220	4.0
macaroni and beef in tomato sauce[a]	10 oz.	60	250	6.0
macaroni and cheese[a]	9 oz.	250	290	9.0
macaroni and cheese[b]	6 oz.	200	250	13.0
macaroni and cheese[d]	9 oz.	250	280	6.0
macaroni and cheese[f]	9 oz.	150	280	6.0
macaroni and cheese nacho[f]	9 oz.	200	280	5.0
mesquite chicken dinner[f]	10.5 oz.	60	300	3.0
nacho grande chicken enchiladas[d]	9.0 oz.	300	280	8.0
noodles Romanoff, Michelini's International Dinners	8 oz.	300	370	20.0
pan pizza, Pappalo's Pillsbury[c]	1/5 pizza	250	320	12.0
pasta Italiano[e]	8.0 oz.	60	160	2.0

	Serving	Calcium (mg)	Calories	Fat (g)
ENTREES AND MEALS, *continued*				
pasta shells, cheese w/tomato sauce[b]	9¼ oz.	350	300	13.0
pasta shells w/tomato sauce[f]	12 oz.	400	330	3.0
pasta w/shrimp and vegetable dinner[f]	12.5 oz.	60	270	4.0
pizza, cheese, Totino's	1/2 pizza	250	290	10.0
pizza, deluxe combo[d]	7.05 oz.	600	320	8.0
pizza, pepperoni[d]	6.08 oz.	350	320	8.0
pizza, pepperoni/sausage, Totino's	1/2 pizza	200	370	17.0
pizza, supreme, Tombstone Light	1/2 pizza	150	190	6.0
pizza, vegetable, Tombstone Light	1/2 pizza	150	170	5.0
ravioli Florentine[g]	8.5 oz.	150	130	1.0
rigatoni bake w/meat sauce and cheese[a]	9¾ oz.	200	250	8.0
Risotto Parmesano, Michelini's International Dinners	8 oz.	350	360	20.0
Romanoff supreme[d]	9.0 oz.	150	230	7.0
Salisbury steak dinner[f]	11.5 oz.	60	280	7.0
Salisbury steak w/gravy and scalloped potatoes[a]	9½ oz.	100	240	7.0
sliced turkey breast w/gravy[f]	10.5 oz.	60	270	4.0
spaghetti w/meatballs[a]	9½ oz.	80	290	7.0
spaghetti w/meatballs[b]	12⅝ oz.	100	440	16.0
spaghetti w/meat sauce[d]	10 oz.	60	240	7.0
stuffed shells, legume	11 oz.	200	240	11.0
Swedish meatballs, Weight Watchers	9 oz.	100	270	8.0
Swedish meatballs in gravy w/ parsley noodles[b]	9¼ oz.	60	420	21.0
three-cheese rotini[d]	9 oz.	250	270	8.0
tortellini, cheese, in Alfredo sauce[b]	8⅞ oz.	400	580	37.0

	Serving	Calcium (mg)	Calories	Fat (g)
ENTREES AND MEALS, *continued*				
tortellini, cheese, w/tomato sauce[b]	9¼ oz.	300	360	16.0
tuna lasagna w/spinach noodles and vegetables[a]	9¾ oz.	200	240	7.0
tuna noodle casserole[b]	10 oz.	150	280	15.0
turkey Dijon[a]	11 oz.	150	260	6.0
turkey pie[b]	10 oz.	100	410	24.0
turkey tetrazzini[b]	10 oz.	100	400	23.0
veal patty Parmigiana[e]	8.2 oz.	150	150	4.0
vegetable lasagna[b]	10½ oz.	300	430	23.0
vegetable primavera baked potato[d]	11.15 oz.	300	320	1.0
Welsh rarebit[b]	5 oz.	350	270	20.0
zucchini lasagna[a]	11 oz.	150	260	6.0

[a] *Stouffer's Lean Cuisine*

[b] *Stouffer's*

[c] *Average values for all varieties*

[d] *Weight Watchers*

[e] *Weight Watchers Ultimate 200*

[f] *Healthy Choice*

[g] *Weight Watchers Smart Ones*

[h] *Chef America*

FAST FOODS
Arby's

	Serving	Calcium (mg)	Calories	Fat (g)
bacon cheddar deluxe	1	110	512	31.5
beef 'n cheddar	1	150	508	26.5
biscuit, plain	1	100	280	14.9
broccoli 'n cheddar baked potato	1	100	417	17.9
cheddar fries	1 order	80	399	21.9

	Serving	Calcium (mg)	Calories	Fat (g)
FAST FOODS, *continued*				
chef salad w/o dressing	1	170	205	9.5
chicken breast fillet	1	60	445	22.5
chicken club	1	180	503	27.0
chicken cordon bleu	1	170	518	27.1
chicken, grilled, deluxe	1	70	430	19.9
croissant, ham and cheese	1	150	345	20.7
croissant, mushroom and cheese	1	200	493	37.7
egg platter	1	60	460	24.0
fish fillet	1	90	526	27.0
French dip 'n Swiss	1	270	429	19.0
garden salad	1	160	117	5.2
ham 'n cheese	1	170	355	14.2
Italian sub	1	410	671	38.8
mushroom 'n cheese baked potato	1	250	515	26.7
Philly beef 'n Swiss	1	290	467	25.3
polar swirl desserts[a]	11.6 oz.	250	500	20.0
roast beef deluxe, light	1	130	294	10.0
roast beef, regular	1	60	383	18.2
roast beef sub	1	410	623	32.0
roast chicken deluxe, light	1	130	276	7.0
roast chicken salad w/o dressing	1	170	204	7.2
roast turkey deluxe, light	1	130	260	6.0
shake, chocolate	12 oz.	250	451	11.6
shake, vanilla	11 oz.	300	330	11.5
soup, clam chowder	8 oz.	150	193	10.0
soup, cream of broccoli	8 oz.	270	166	7.2
soup, potato w/bacon	8 oz.	170	184	8.8
soup, Wisconsin cheese	8 oz.	290	281	18.0
tuna sub	1	420	663	37.0
turkey sub	1	400	486	19.0

[a] *Average values for all flavors*

	Serving	Calcium (mg)	Calories	Fat (g)
FAST FOODS, *continued*				
Burger King				
cheeseburger	1	102	300	14.0
cheeseburger, double w/bacon	1	200	470	28.0
chef salad w/o dressing	1	160	273	9.0
chicken sandwich	1	79	620	32.0
croissandwich, bacon or ham, egg, and cheese	1	136	532	22.5
croissandwich, sausage, egg, and cheese	1	145	534	40.0
garden salad w/o dressing	1	150	223	5.0
French toast sticks	1 order	60	440	24.0
lemon pie	1 slice	100	290	8.0
onion rings	1 regular serving	110	339	19.0
shakes, chocolate/vanilla	1 medium	310	330	10.0
shake, strawberry (syrup added)	1 medium	310	394	10.0
Snickers ice cream bar	1	60	220	14.0
Whopper	1	80	570	31.0
Whopper Jr. w/cheese	1	105	350	19.0
Whopper double, w/cheese	1	250	890	55.0
Whopper w/cheese	1	210	660	48.0
Dairy Queen				
banana split	1	300	510	11.0
barbecue beef sandwich	1	100	225	9.0
Blizzard, Heath	1 regular	400	820	36.0
breaded chicken fillet w/ cheese	1	100	480	25.0
Breeze, Heath	1 regular	500	680	21.0
Buster Bar	1	300	450	29.0
cone	1 large	200	340	10.0

	Serving	Calcium (mg)	Calories	Fat (g)
FAST FOODS, *continued*				
cone	1 regular	150	230	7.0
cone, chocolate dipped	1 regular	300	330	16.0
Dilly Bar	1	250	210	13.0
DQ sandwich	1	60	140	4.0
fish fillet sandwich w/cheese	1	100	420	21.0
frozen cake	1 slice	150	380	18.0
frozen yogurt cone	1 regular	200	180	<1.0
frozen yogurt cup	1 regular	250	170	<1.0
garden salad w/o dressing	1	250	200	13.0
grilled chicken sandwich	1	60	300	8.0
hamburger w/cheese	1	150	365	18.0
hot dog w/cheese	1	100	330	21.0
hot fudge brownie delight	1	300	710	29.0
Peanut Buster Parfait	1	350	710	32.0
shake[a]	1 regular	400	530	14.0
sundae, chocolate	1 regular	150	300	7.0
Domino's				
pepperoni pizza, 12"	2 slices	200	437	14.5
veggie pizza, 12"	2 slices	200	408	11.0
Kentucky Fried Chicken				
beans, baked	1 serving	54	105	1.2
biscuit, buttermilk	1	95	235	11.7
chicken, breast, original recipe	1	68	267	16.5
chicken, thigh, original recipe	1	65	294	19.7
McDonald's				
Big Mac	1	250	500	26.0
biscuit, w/bacon, egg, and cheese	1	200	440	26.0
biscuit w/sausage	1	80	420	28.0
biscuit w/spread	1	74	260	12.7

	Serving	Calcium (mg)	Calories	Fat (g)
FAST FOODS, *continued*				
cheeseburger	1	200	305	13.0
chef salad w/o dressing	1	150	170	9.0
chicken fajita	1	80	185	8.0
Egg McMuffin	1	250	280	11.0
English muffin w/spread	1	150	170	4.0
Filet-O-Fish	1	150	370	18.0
frozen yogurt cone	3 oz.	100	105	1.0
frozen yogurt sundae	6 oz.	200	270	2.8
frozen yogurt sundae, hot fudge	6 oz.	250	240	3.0
frozen yogurt sundae, strawberry	6 oz.	200	210	1.1
hamburger	1	100	255	9.0
hot cakes w/margarine and syrup	1 order	100	440	12.0
McChicken sandwich	1	150	370	20.0
Quarter Pounder	1	150	410	20.0
Quarter Pounder w/cheese	1	300	510	28.0
scrambled eggs	1 order	60	140	10.0
shake[a]	10.4 oz.	300	310	1.5
Pizza Hut				
pizza, cheese, family size	2 slices	300	380	14.0
pizza, cheese, personal size	1	350	500	18.0
pizza, pepperoni, family size	2 slices	300	430	18.0
pizza, pepperoni, personal size	1	350	550	22.0
Subway				
blue cheese dressing	2 oz.	62	322	28.6
BMT salad w/o dressing	1 regular	162	635	51.9
BMT sub, Italian roll	1	195	982	55.3
cold cut combo salad w/o dressing	1 regular	193	506	36.5

	Serving	Calcium (mg)	Calories	Fat (g)
FAST FOODS, *continued*				
cold cut combo sub, Italian roll	1	390	853	40.0
ham and cheese salad w/o dressing	1 regular	145	296	17.7
ham and cheese sub, Italian roll	1	172	643	17.9
meatball sub, Italian roll	1	219	918	43.7
roast beef salad w/o dressing	1 regular	80	340	19.7
roast beef sub, Italian roll	1	179	689	23.2
seafood and crab salad	1 regular	259	639	53.5
seafood and crab sub	1	266	986	56.9
seafood and lobster salad	1 regular	154	597	49.4
seafood and lobster sub, Italian roll	1	187	944	52.7
spicy Italian salad w/o dressing	1 regular	160	696	59.5
spicy Italian sub, Italian roll	1	192	1043	63.0
steak and cheese sub, Italian roll	1	189	765	31.5
Subway club salad w/o dressing	1 regular	147	346	18.7
Subway club sub, Italian roll	1	180	693	22.2
turkey breast salad w/o dressing	1 regular	145	297	15.8
turkey breast sub, Italian roll	1	178	645	19.3
tuna salad	1 regular	500	756	68.0
tuna salad sub, Italian roll	1	530	1103	71.7
veggies and cheese salad w/o dressing	1 regular	139	188	13.7
veggies and cheese sub, Italian roll	1	172	535	17.2
Taco Bell				
burrito, bean	1	190	357	14.0
burrito, beef	1	150	493	21.0
burrito, chicken	1	110	334	12.0

	Serving	Calcium (mg)	Calories	Fat (g)
FAST FOODS, *continued*				
chilito	1	270	383	18.0
Mexican pizza	1	257	575	37.0
Mexmelt, beef	1	270	266	15.0
Mexmelt, chicken	1	250	257	15.0
nachos bellgrande	1 order	297	649	35.0
nachos supreme	1 order	260	367	27.0
pintos and cheese	1	156	190	9.0
soft taco	1	116	225	12.0
soft taco, chicken	1	80	213	10.0
soft taco, supreme	1	142	272	16.0
taco	1	84	183	11.0
taco bellgrande	1	182	335	23.0
taco salad	1	320	905	61.0
taco salad w/o shell	1	280	484	31.0
tostada	1	180	243	11.0
Wendy's				
baked potato w/bacon and cheese	1	100	510	17.0
baked potato w/broccoli and cheese	1	100	450	14.0
baked potato w/cheese	1	300	550	24.0
baked potato w/chili and cheese	1	300	600	25.0
baked potato w/sour cream and chives	1	80	370	6.0
Big Classic	1	150	480	23.0
Caesar side salad	1	80	160	6.0
cheeseburger, Jr.	1	150	320	13.0
cheeseburger, deluxe, Jr.	1	200	390	20.0
chicken club sandwich	1	100	520	25.0
chicken sandwich	1	100	450	20.0
chili	8 oz.	80	190	6.0
fish sandwich	1	100	460	25.0

	Serving	Calcium (mg)	Calories	Fat (g)
FAST FOOD, *continued*				
Frosty	1 small	300	340	10.0
Frosty	1 medium	400	460	13.0
Frosty	1 large	500	570	17.0
garden salad w/o dressing	1	200	110	5.0
grilled chicken salad w/o dressing	1	200	200	8.0
grilled chicken sandwich	1	100	290	7.0
hamburger, single	1	100	350	15.0
shredded cheese, imitation (salad bar)	2 T	100	50	4.0
side salad w/o dressing	1	100	60	3.0
taco salad w/o dressing	1	450	640	30.0
FISH, SHELLFISH, AND CRUSTACEA				
anchovies, canned	3 oz.	125	111	4.1
bass, freshwater, baked	3 oz.	68	97	3.1
clams, canned	3 oz.	78	126	1.7
clams, breaded and fried	3 oz.	54	171	9.5
cod, dried and salted	3 oz.	136	246	2.0
crab, Alaskan king, cooked by moist heat	3 oz.	50	82	1.3
crab, blue, cooked by moist heat	3 oz.	88	87	1.5
crab cakes	1 cake	63	93	4.5
lobster, northern, cooked by moist heat	3 oz.	52	83	0.5
mackerel, jack, canned	1 cup	458	296	12.0
ocean perch, Atlantic, baked	3 oz.	117	103	1.8
oysters, eastern, cooked by moist heat	12 medium	76	117	4.2
oysters, eastern, breaded and fried	6 medium	53	167	10.7
pike, northern, baked	3 oz.	62	96	0.8

	Serving	Calcium (mg)	Calories	Fat (g)
FISH, SHELLFISH, AND CRUSTACEA, *continued*				
pike, walleye, baked	3 oz.	94	79	1.0
pollack, Atlantic, baked	3 oz.	51	78	0.8
salmon, chum, end w/bone[a]	3 oz.	212[a]	120	4.7
salmon, pink, end w/bone[a]	3 oz.	181[a]	118	5.1
salmon, sockeye, end w/ bone[a]	3 oz.	203[a]	130	6.2
sardines, Atlantic, canned in soybean oil[a]	2 sardines	92[a]	68	4.6
shrimp, baked	4 oz.	55	100	1.1
shrimp, breaded and fried	3 oz.	57	206	10.4
shrimp, canned	3 oz.	50	102	1.7
smelt, Atlantic, canned	4–5 medium	358	200	13.5
smelt, rainbow, baked	3 oz.	65	106	2.6
sole, baked	3.5 oz.	61	68	0.5
trout, rainbow, baked	3 oz.	73	129	3.7
whiting, baked	3 oz.	53	98	1.4

[a]*If bones are discarded, calcium is greatly reduced.*

FROZEN SIDE DISHES				
corn soufflé[b]	6 oz.	60	240	11.0
creamed spinach[b]	4½ oz.	100	190	16.0
fettuccini Alfredo[b]	5 oz.	150	245	14.0
green bean mushroom casserole[b]	4¾ oz.	80	160	10.0
noodles Romanoff[a]	5¾ oz.	100	130	6.0
potato, broccoli and cheese, Ore-Ida	5⅗ oz.	150	160	4.0
potato, cheese and salsa, Ore-Ida	5⅗ oz.	150	160	4.0

Note: A sampling of frozen dinners has been included to familiarize you with meals providing a minimum of 50 milligrams of calcium. Most frozen entree lines offer meals supplying calcium.

	Serving	Calcium (mg)	Calories	Fat (g)
FROZEN SIDE DISHES, *continued*				
potatoes au gratin[b]	5¾ oz.	100	130	6.0
potato, twice baked, Ore-Ida	5 oz.	60	180	6.0
spinach soufflé[c]	6 oz.	150	220	15.0

[a] *Stouffer's Lean Cuisine*

[b] *Stouffer's*

[c] *Average values for all varieties*

HOMEMADE ENTREES				
beef, dried, chipped, cooked creamed	1 cup	257	377	25.2
chicken a la king	1 cup	127	468	34.3
chop suey	1 cup	60	300	17.0
eggplant Parmesan	1 cup	310	356	24.0
fettuccini Alfredo	1 cup	252	461	29.7
green pepper stuffed w/beef and crumbs	1	78	315	10.2
lasagna w/beef and cheese	1 piece	244	400	19.8
lobster Newburg	1 cup	218	485	26.5
macaroni and cheese	1 cup	362	430	22.2
oyster stew	1 cup (6 oysters)	274	233	15.4
quiche, plain	1 slice	188	312	17.6
salmon patty	3.5 oz.	78	239	12.4
spaghetti w/meatballs and tomato sauce	1 cup	124	332	11.7
spaghetti w/tomato sauce	1 cup	80	260	8.8
tortellini, cheese, w/tomato sauce	1 cup	133	363	10.4
tortellini, meat, w/tomato sauce	1 cup	93	350	10.4
veal Parmigiana	1 cup	198	485	25.5
Welsh rarebit	1 cup	582	415	31.6

	Serving	Calcium (mg)	Calories	Fat (g)
FRUIT AND FRUIT JUICES/ DRINKS				
cherimoya	1 medium	126	515	2.2
citrus punch, Sunny Delight plus calcium	6 oz.	200	90	<1.0
currants, zante, dried[a]	1/2 cup	62	204	0.2
elderberries, raw	1 cup	55	105	0.7
figs, dried	10 figs	269	477	2.2
grapefruit juice cocktail, Citrus Hill plus calcium	6 oz.	200	70	<1.0
jujube, dried	3.5 oz.	79	287	1.1
mulberries, raw	1 cup	66	67	0.6
orange juice, Minute Maid plus calcium	6 oz.	200	90	<1.0
orange, navel	1 medium	56	65	0.1
papaya	1 medium	72	117	0.4
pear, dried	10 halves	59	459	1.1
prickly pear	1 medium	58	42	0.5
raisins, golden, seedless	2/3 cup	53	302	0.5
roselle	1 cup	123	28	0.4
sapote	1 medium	88	301	1.4
tamarind	1 cup	89	287	0.7

[a]*Dried black Corinth grapes*

MEATS, LUNCHEON				
frankfurter, turkey, Louis Rich	1 frank	61	103	8.5
frankfurter, turkey w/cheese, Oscar Mayer	1 frank	55	108	8.3

MEAT SPREADS				
chicken, canned, Swanson	1.02 oz.	62	60	3.9
ham and cheese, Oscar Mayer	1 oz.	51	66	5.1

	Serving	Calcium (mg)	Calories	Fat (g)
MILK				
buttermilk, cultured, 1% fat	8 oz.	300	100	2.0
buttermilk, cultured, 1½% fat	8 oz.	300	120	4.0
buttermilk, dry	1 T	77	25	0.4
Calcimilk (lactose-reduced)	8 oz.	500	90	<1.0
condensed, sweetened, canned	1 oz.	108	123	3.3
evaporated, lowfat, canned	4 oz.	318	110	3.0
evaporated, skim, canned	4 oz.	368	100	0.4
evaporated, whole, canned	4 oz.	329	169	9.5
goat milk	8 oz.	326	168	10.1
Lactaid (lactose-reduced), nonfat	8 oz.	300	90	0.0
lowfat, 1% fat	8 oz.	300	100	2.0
lowfat, 2% fat	8 oz.	297	121	4.7
sheep milk	8 oz.	474	264	17.2
skim	8 oz.	302	86	0.4
skim, dry	1/4 cup	377	109	0.2
whole, 3.5%	8 oz.	288	150	8.6
whole, dry	1/4 cup	292	159	10.1
MILK BEVERAGES				
Alba, chocolate flavor, nonfat dry milk in water	8 oz.	310	80	1.0
chocolate milk, 1% fat	8 oz.	287	158	2.5
chocolate milk, 2% fat	8 oz.	284	179	5.0
chocolate milk, 3.5% fat	8 oz.	280	208	8.5
cocoa, hot, prepared w/6 oz. water, from mix (rich chocolate flavor)	4 heaping tsp.	60	110	1.0
cocoa, hot, diet, prepared w/ water, Carnation/Alba	1 packet	80	25	0.0
cocoa, hot, Carnation sugar-free mix, prepared w/6 oz. water	4 heaping tsp.	150	50	0.0
cocoa, hot, Weight Watchers, prepared w/6 oz. water	1 packet	300	60	0.0

	Serving	Calcium (mg)	Calories	Fat (g)
MILK BEVERAGES, *continued*				
eggnog, nonalcoholic	8 oz.	330	342	19.0
Fit 'N Frosty, Alba, chocolate, prepared w/water	1 packet	250	70	0.0
Fit 'N Frosty, Alba, double fudge, prepared w/water	1 packet	350	60	0.0
Fit 'N Frosty, Alba, vanilla, prepared w/water	1 packet	300	70	0.0
instant breakfast, Carnation, all flavors	1 packet	100	130	1.0
instant breakfast, Carnation, prepared w/2% milk	1 packet + 8 oz. milk	400	250	6.0
instant breakfast, Carnation sugar-free, all flavors	1 packet	100	70	1.0
instant breakfast, Carnation sugar-free, prepared w/2% milk	1 packet + 8 oz. milk	400	190	6.0
malted milk	8 oz.	347	236	9.9
milkshake, chocolate, thick	1 avg.	396	356	8.1
milkshake, vanilla, thick	1 avg.	457	350	9.5
Ovaltine powder	3/4 oz.	80	80	0.0
shake mix, Weight Watchers, chocolate/orange	1 packet	300	70	<1.0
Vitamite (lactose-free)	8 oz.	250	110	5.0
YOGURT (*average values for various brands*)				
coffee/vanilla flavor, lowfat	8 oz.	300	200	2.6
fruit flavored, low-fat	8 oz.	350	240	2.8
fruit flavored, nonfat	6 oz.	250	150	0.0
fruit flavored, nonfat, sugar-free	8 oz.	350	100	0.0
plain, nonfat	8 oz.	400	110	0.0
plain, low-fat	8 oz.	400	140	4.0
vanilla flavored, nonfat, sugar-free	8 oz.	350	100	0.0

	Serving	Calcium (mg)	Calories	Fat (g)
NUTS, NUT PRODUCTS, AND SEEDS				
almond meal, partially defatted	1 oz.	120	116	5.2
almond paste	1 oz.	65	127	7.7
almonds, blanched, Blue Diamond	1 oz.	73	174	14.4
almonds, cheese, Blue Diamond	1 oz.	102	156	12.5
almonds, dry roasted, hickory smoke, Blue Diamond	1 oz.	117	166	15.0
almonds, onion and garlic, Blue Diamond	1 oz.	125	160	13.6
beechnuts, dried	1 oz.	50	164	14.2
Brazil nuts	1 oz.	50	186	18.8
coconut water[a]	8 oz.	58	46	0.5
hazelnuts, Filberts, dry roasted	1 oz.	55	188	18.8
sesame butter (tahini)	1 T.	64	89	8.1
sesame seeds, whole, toasted	1 oz.	281	161	13.6
soybean nuts, dry roasted	1/2 cup	232	387	18.6

[a] *Liquid from coconuts, not the "milk"*

	Serving	Calcium (mg)	Calories	Fat (g)
SALAD DRESSING				
Slimfast salad dressing (*average values for all flavors*)	1 T	100	6	<1.0
SAUCES/DIPS				
Alfredo sauce, refrigerated, Fresh Chef	4 oz.	202	298	26.8
curry sauce, from mix	1/4 packet prep.	152	84	4.6
hot fudge topping, Smucker's Light	2 T	80	70	0.0
hummus	1/2 cup	62	210	10.4
pesto sauce, refrigerated, Fresh Chef	1 oz.	98	155	14.6

	Serving	Calcium (mg)	Calories	Fat (g)
SAUCES/DIPS, *continued*				
sour cream sauce, from mix	1/4 packet prep.	68	64	3.8
spaghetti sauce, Ragu Fino Italian Parmesan	4 oz.	60	90	3.0
Stroganoff sauce, from mix	1/4 packet prep.	141	73	2.9
white sauce, from mix	1/4 packet prep.	265	151	8.4
SNACK FOODS				
cheese curls, Slimfast[b]	1 oz.	100	110	3.0
cheese straws[a]	10 pieces	155	272	17.9
cheese/toast crackers w/ peanut butter[a]	1.5 oz.	60	210	10.0
FI-BAR	1 bar	60	130	4.0
FI-BAR a.m.	1 bar	100	150	4.0
pretzels, Slimfast[b]	1 oz.	100	100	1.0
popcorn, Slimfast[b]	1/2 oz.	100	60	2.0
popcorn, caramel, Slimfast[b]	1 oz.	100	120	1.0
snack bar, Slimfast[b]	1 oz.	150	110	4.0
wheat crackers w/peanut butter[a]	1.5 oz.	60	205	10.0
tortilla chips, baked, Tostitos	1.5 oz.	60	195	3.0
tortilla chips, nacho/taco flavor, Doritos	1.5 oz.	60	210	10.5

[a] *Average for all flavors*

[b] *Vitamin-fortified*

SOUPS, CANNED, CONDENSED, PREPARED W/ MILK				
clam chowder, New England	1 cup	187	163	6.6
cheese	1 cup	288	230	14.6
cream of asparagus	1 cup	175	161	8.2
cream of celery	1 cup	186	165	9.7

	Serving	Calcium (mg)	Calories	Fat (g)
SOUPS, CANNED, CONDENSED, PREPARED W/MILK, *continued*				
cream of chicken	1 cup	180	191	11.5
cream of mushroom	1 cup	187	203	13.6
cream of potato	1 cup	166	148	6.5
oyster stew	1 cup	167	134	7.9
tomato	1 cup	159	160	6.0
SOUPS, CANNED, CONDENSED, PREPARED W/ WATER				
bean w/bacon	1 cup	81	173	5.9
bean w/franks	1 cup	86	187	7.0
cheese	1 cup	142	155	10.5
nacho cheese	1 cup	78	105	7.2
SOUPS, CANNED, READY-TO-SERVE				
bean, Campbell's	7.5 oz.	72	143	3.9
bean w/ham, Campbell's	1 cup	79	231	8.5
beef ravioli Romano, Chunky Campbell's	9.49 oz.	64	231	8.3
beef w/noodles, Stroganoff style, Chunky Campbell's	10.76 oz.	76	300	14.1
black bean and vegetable, Health Valley	7.5 oz.	60	70	0.0
chili, beef, Chunky Campbell's	9.74 oz.	61	256	5.7
clam chowder, New England, Chunky Campbell's	10.76 oz.	63	162	4.0
fisherman chowder, Chunky Campbell's	9.49 oz.	67	229	12.2
lentil and carrots, Health Valley	7.5 oz.	60	70	0.0
lentil, Home Cookin', Campbell's	10.76 oz.	71	150	4.3
tortilla, Chunky Campbell's	10.76 oz.	101	293	9.6

	Serving	Calcium (mg)	Calories	Fat (g)
SOUPS, DRIED MIX, PREPARED W/WATER				
Slimfast instant soups	1 envelope	100	45	<1.0
SPECIAL DIETARY FOODS				
Dynatrim, Centrum, prepared w/8 oz. 1% milk	1 scoop	500	220	4.0
Ensure, liquid nutrition	8 oz.	125	250	8.8
Ensure Plus, liquid nutrition	8 oz.	167	355	12.6
figurine diet bar, Pillsbury	1 bar	60	100	5.0
Nutrament drink, chocolate/ vanilla	12 oz.	350	360	10.0
Slender bars, Carnation	2 bars	250	270	1.6
Slender liquid diet meal, canned, Carnation	10 oz.	250	220	4.0
Slimfast powder, prepared w/ 8 oz. skim milk, café mocha/ chocolate royale	1 scoop	500	210	1.0
Slimfast powder, prepared w/ 8 oz. skim milk, vanilla/ chocolate/strawberry	1 scoop	450	190	1.0
Slimfast powder, prepared w/ 8 oz. orange juice	1 scoop	350	200	<1.0
VEGETABLES AND VEGETABLE PRODUCTS (starchy beans and soy products included)				
adzuki beans, boiled	1 cup	66	294	0.6
amaranth, boiled	1/2 cup	138	14	0.1
beans, refried, canned	7.5 oz.	60	250	11.0
beet greens, boiled	1/2 cup	82	20	0.1

Tip: Homemade soups made from meat or poultry bones can be a rich source of calcium if a small amount of vinegar is added to the soup. The acid from the vinegar pulls out the calcium from the bones.

	Serving	Calcium (mg)	Calories	Fat (g)
VEGETABLES AND VEGETABLE PRODUCTS, *continued*				
black turtle beans, canned	1 cup	103	241	0.6
bok choy	1 cup	160	20	0.2
broad beans, canned	1 cup	62	183	0.6
broccoli, boiled	1/2 cup	89	23	0.2
broccoli w/cheese sauce, Birds Eye	1/2 cup	109	116	6.2
brussels sprouts w/cheese sauce, Birds Eye	1/2 cup	77	113	5.6
cassava, raw	3.5 oz.	91	120	0.4
cauliflower w/cheese sauce, Birds Eye	1/2 cup	83	114	6.1
chard, Swiss, chopped, boiled	1/2 cup	51	18	0.1
chick peas, canned, boiled	1 cup	78	285	2.7
chickory greens, raw, chopped	1/2 cup	90	21	0.3
collard greens, frozen, boiled, chopped	1/2 cup	179	31	0.4
cranberry beans, canned	1 cup	87	216	0.7
dandelion greens, boiled	1/2 cup	73	17	0.3
great northern beans, canned	1 cup	130	180	0.2
kale, frozen, boiled, chopped	1/2 cup	90	20	0.3
kidney beans, canned, boiled	1 cup	62	216	0.6
lima beans, frozen, boiled	1 cup	50	188	0.6
mustard greens, frozen, boiled, chopped	1/2 cup	75	14	0.2
navy beans, canned, boiled	1 cup	123	296	1.1
okra, frozen, boiled, sliced	1/2 cup	88	34	0.3
onions, small w/cream sauce, Birds Eye	1/2 cup	55	100	5.9
pinto beans, canned, boiled	1 cup	89	186	0.8
potato, mashed from flakes, made w/milk	1/2 cup	52	118	5.9
potatoes, au gratin, from mix, prepared w/milk	1/6 of 5.5 oz. pkg.	114	127	5.6
potatoes, scalloped, homemade	1/2 cup	70	105	4.5

	Serving	Calcium (mg)	Calories	Fat (g)
VEGETABLES AND VEGETABLE PRODUCTS, *continued*				
radish, oriental (daikon and Chinese), dried	1/2 cup	365	157	0.4
rhubarb, frozen, cooked, sweetened	1/2 cup	174	139	0.1
rhubarb, frozen, raw	1 cup	266	29	0.2
seaweed, agar, raw	3.5 oz.	54	26	0.0
seaweed, kelp (kombu), raw	3.5 oz.	168	43	0.6
seaweed, wakame, raw	3.5 oz.	150	45	0.6
SOYBEAN PRODUCTS				
miso	1/2 cup	92	284	8.4
natto	1/2 cup	191	187	9.7
tempeh	1/2 cup	77	165	6.4
tofu, raw (soft)	1/2 cup	130	94	5.9
tofu, raw (firm)	1/2 cup	258	183	11.0
soybeans, green, boiled	1/2 cup	131	127	5.8
spinach, boiled	1/2 cup	122	21	0.2
spinach, creamed, frozen, Pillsbury	1/2 cup	130	80	2.9
spinach w/butter sauce, frozen, Pillsbury	1/2 cup	207	60	1.5
turnip greens, boiled, chopped	1/2 cup	99	15	0.2
wax beans, cut, canned, Joan of Arc	1/2 cup	87	25	0.2
white beans, boiled	1 cup	161	249	0.6
MISCELLANEOUS				
baking powder, Calumet	1 tsp.	241	3	0.0
rennin (salt, starch, rennin enzyme)	1 packet	386	12	0.1
yeast, brewer's	1 oz.	60	80	0.3

Recommended Reading and References

Bergfeld, Wilma F., M.D., F.A.C.P., and Shelagh Ryan Masline. *A Woman Doctor's Guide to Skin Care*. New York: Hyperion, 1995.

Carrico, Mara, and the Editors of *Yoga Journal*. *Yoga Basics: The Essential Beginner's Guide to Yoga for a Lifetime of Health and Fitness*. New York: Henry Holt and Company, 1997.

Frawley, David, M.D., and Vasant Lad, M.D. *The Yoga of Herbs*. Twin Lakes, Wis.: Lotus Press, 1986.

Greer, Germaine. *The Change: Women, Aging, and the Menopause*. New York: Alfred A. Knopf, 1992.

Hufnagel, Vicki, M.D., with Susan K. Golant. *No More Hysterectomies*. New York: Plume, 1989.

Jacobowitz, Ruth S. *150 Most-Asked Questions About Menopause: What Women Really Want to Know*. New York: William Morrow/Hearst Books, 1993.

Jacobowitz, Ruth S. *150 Most-Asked Questions About Midlife Sex, Love, and Intimacy*. New York: William Morrow/Hearst Books, 1995.

Jacobowitz, Ruth S. *150 Most-Asked Questions About Osteoporosis*. New York: William Morrow/Hearst Books, 1993.

Lark, Susan M., M.D. *The Estrogen Decision Self Help Book*. Berkeley: Celestial Arts, 1993.

Love, Susan M., M.D., and Karen Lindsay. *Dr. Susan Love's Hormone Book*. New York: Random House, 1997.

Luchetti, Cathy. *The Hot Flash Cookbook*. San Francisco: Chronicle, 1997.

Nelson, Miriam E., Ph.D. *Strong Women Stay Young*. New York: Bantam, 1997.

Northrup, Christiane, M.D. *Women's Bodies, Women's Wisdom*. New York: Bantam, 1994.

Schiff, Issac, M.D., with Ann B. Parson. *Menopause*. New York: Times Books, 1996.

Utian, Wulf H., M.D., Ph.D., and Ruth S. Jacobowitz. *Managing Your Menopause*. New York: Simon and Schuster/Fireside, 1990.

Vliet, Elizabeth Lee, M.D. *Screaming to Be Heard*. New York: M. Evans and Company, 1995.

Weed, Susun. *Menopausal Years: The Wise Woman Way*. Woodstock, N.Y.: Ash Tree Publishing, 1995.

Your Health. Published monthly by Globe International Inc., 5401 NW Broken Sound Blvd., Boca Raton, FL 33487. Subscription $19.95 per year. Published 12 times per year.

Other Professional Sources

"A comparative study of safety and efficacy of continuous low-dose oestradiol released from a vaginal ring compared with conjugated equine oestrogen vaginal cream in the treatment of postmenopausal urogenital atrophy." *British Journal of Obstetrics and Gynaecology* 103 (April 1996): 351–358.

Ambrosone, C. B., et al. "Cigarette Smoking, N-acetyltransferase 2 genetic polymorphisms, and breast cancer risk." *Journal of the American Medical Association.* November 13, 1996: 1494–1501.

American Heart Association. "About Women, Heart Disease, and Stroke." *1998 Heart and Stroke Statistical Update* (1998): 2.

Andrews, William C., M.D. "The Transitional Years and Beyond." *Obstetrics and Gynecology* 85 (January 1995): 1–5.

Angier, Natalie. "Theorists See Evolutionary Advantages in Menopause." *New York Times,* September 16, 1997: B-9.

Baylis, Francoise, Ph.D. "Access to Health Care for Women." *New England Journal of Medicine* 336, no. 25 (1997): 1841.

Belchetz, Paul E. "Hormonal Treatment of Postmenopausal Women." *New England Journal of Medicine* 330, no. 15 (April 14, 1994): 1062.

Birge, Stanley J., M.D. "Is There a Role for Estrogen Replacement Therapy in the Prevention and Treatment of Dementia?" *Journal of the American Geriatrics Society* 44 (July 1996): 865–870.

Black, D. M., et al. "Alendronate Reduces Fractures in Women at Risk." *Journal Watch* 17 (January 15, 1997): 13.

Brinton, L. A., and C. Schairer. "Postmenopausal Hormone-Replacement Therapy — Time for a Reappraisal?" *New England Journal of Medicine* 336 (June 19, 1997): 1821.

Brody, Jane E. "Diet May Be One Reason Complaints about Menopause Are Rare in Asia." *New York Times*, August 27, 1997: B-10.

———. "Hormone Use Helps Women, a Study Finds." *New York Times*, June 19, 1997: A-1.

Brunton, Stephen A., M.D. "Estrogen Replacement Therapy (ERT): Results of a Patient Satisfaction Survey of Women Receiving ERT and Implications for Treatment." *Today's Therapeutic Trends* 14, no. 3 (1996): 119–130.

Barrett-Connor, Elizabeth, M.D. "Risks and Benefits of Replacement Estrogen." *Annual Review of Medicine* 43 (1992): 239–251.

Cagnacci, Angelo, et al. "Depression and Anxiety in Climacteric Women: Role of Hormone Replacement Therapy." *Menopause: The Journal of the North American Menopause Society* 4, no. 4 (1997): 206–211.

Cauley, J. A., et al. "Bone Mineral Density and Risk of Breast Cancer in Older Women: The Study of Osteoporotic Fractures." *Journal of the American Medical Association* 276 (November 6, 1996): 1404–1408.

Chesnut III, Charles H., et al. "Hormone Replacement Therapy in Postmenopausal Women: Urinary N-Telopeptide of Type I Collagen Monitors Therapeutic Effect and Predicts Response of Bone Mineral Density." *American Journal of Medicine* 102 (January 1997): 29–37.

Col, N. F., et al. "Patient-Specific Decisions about Hormone Replacement Therapy in Postmenopausal Women." *Journal of the American Medical Association* 277 (April 9, 1997): 1140–1147.

"Collaborative Group on Hormonal Factors in Breast Cancer. Breast Cancer and Hormone Replacement Therapy: Collaborative Reanalysis of Data from 51 Epidemiological Studies of 52,705 Women with Breast Cancer and 108,411 Women without Breast Cancer." *Lancet* 350 (October 11, 1997): 1047–1059.

Colditz, Graham A., M.B., B.S., et al. "The use of estrogens and progestins and the risk of breast cancer in postmenopausal women." *New England Journal of Medicine* 332, no. 24 (1995): 1589–1639.

Covello, Vincent T., Ph.D. "Women's perceptions of the risks of age-related disease, including breast cancer: A case study." *Center for Risk Communication.* (November 1997).

Delmas, Pierre D., et al. "Effects of Raloxifene on bone mineral density, serum cholesterol concentrations, and uterine endometrium in postmenopausal women." *New England Journal of Medicine* 337, no. 23 (1997): 1641–1648.

DePalma, Anthony. "World Breast Cancer Forum Blames Environmental Ills." *New York Times,* July 19, 1997: Y-4.

Douketis, J. D., et al. "A reevaluation of the risk for venous thromboembolism with the use of oral contraceptives and hormone replacement therapy." *Archives of Internal Medicine* 157 (July 28, 1997): 1522–1530.

Drachman, D. A. et al. "Treatment of Alzheimer's Disease — Searching for a Breakthrough, Settling for Less." *New England Journal of Medicine* 336, no. 17 (April 24, 1997): 1245–1248.

Espeland, M. A., et al. "Effect of postmenopausal hormone therapy on body weight and waist and hip girths." *Journal of Clinical Endocrinology and Metabolism* 82 (May 1997): 1549–1556.

"Estracomb TTS: The Transdermal Therapeutic System for Combined Replacement of Estrogen and Progestin." *Novartis* (formerly *Ciba and Sandoz*).

"Estrogen and Memory." *Journal of the American Medical Association* 279, no. 4 (1998): 262.

"Estrogen Trial Evaluation Impact on Alzheimer's Disease Ends First-Year Recruitment with One-Quarter of Women Needed." *Women's Health Initiative Memory Study,* May 8, 1997.

Ettinger, Bruce, et al. "Continuation of Postmenopausal Hormone Replacement Therapy: Comparison of Cyclic Versus Continuous Combined Schedules." *Menopause* 3, no. 4 (1996): 185–189.

———. "Long-Term Postmenopausal Estrogen Therapy May Be Associated with Increased Risk of Breast Cancer: A Cohort Study." *Menopause* 4, no. 3 (1997): 125–129.

———. "Clinical Trial of Dong Quai for Menopausal Symptoms." *Menopause* 4, no. 4 (1997): 239.

Fries, James F., M.D. "Editorial: Can Preventive Gerontology Be on the Way?" *American Journal of Public Health* 87, no. 10 (1997): 1591–1593.

Fuleihan, G. El-Haji. "Tissue-Specific Estrogens — the Promise for the Future." *New England Journal of Medicine* 337, no. 23 (1997): 1686.

Garber, J. E., and E. Oliva. "A 67-Year Old Woman with Increasing Neurologic Deficits and a History of Breast and Ovarian Cancer." *New England Journal of Medicine* 337, no. 11 (1997): 770–779.

Ghali, W. A., et al. "Menopausal Hormone Therapy: Physician Awareness of Patient Attitudes." *American Journal of Medicine* 103 (July 1997): 3–10.

Good, William R., Ph.D., et al. "Double-Masked, Multicenter Study of an Estradiol Matrix Transdermal Delivery System (Alora) Versus Placebo in Postmenopausal Women Experiencing Menopausal Symptoms." *Clinical Therapeutics* 18, no. 6 (1996): 1093.

Grady, Deborah, M.D., M.P.H., et al. "Hormone Therapy to Prevent Disease and Prolong Life in Postmenopausal Women." *Annals of Internal Medicine* 117, no. 12 (1992): 1016–1037.

Grady, Denise. "Study Favors Monounsaturated Fat." *New York Times*, January 13, 1998: B-2.

Greenwood, Sadja, M.D., M.P.H., et al. "Focus on OTC 'Naturals.' " *Menopause Management* 6, no. 4 (1997): 6–15.

Grodstein, Francine, Sc.D., et al. "Postmenopausal Hormone Therapy and Mortality." *New England Journal of Medicine* 336, no. 25 (1997): 1769–1775.

———. "Postmenopausal Estrogen and Progestin Use and the Risk of Cardiovascular Disease." *New England Journal of Medicine* 335, no. 7 (1996): 453–461.

———. "Postmenopausal Hormone Use and Tooth Loss: A Prospective Study." *Journal of the American Dental Association* 127 (March 1996): 370–377.

"Ginkgo Biloba Relieves Some Vascular Problems." *Better Nutrition for Today's Living*, November 1993: 12.

Henderson, Victor W., M.D. "The Epidemiology of Estrogen Replacement Therapy and Alzheimer's Disease." *Neurology*, May 1977: 827–835.

Henriksson, Lars, M.D., Ph.D., et al. "A One-Year Multicenter Study of Efficacy and Safety of a Continuous, Low-Dose, Estradiol-Releasing Vaginal Ring (Estring) in Postmenopausal Women with Symptoms and Signs of Urogenital Aging." *American Journal of Obstetrics and Gynecology* 174 (1996): 85–92.

"Hormone Replacement Therapy." *ACOG Technical Bulletin* no. 166 (April 1992).

Hoskins, David, M.D., et al. "Prevention of Bone Loss with Alendronate in Postmenopausal Women Under 60 Years of Age." *New England Journal of Medicine* 338, no. 9 (1998): 485–492.

Huang, Zhiping, M.D., Ph.D., et al. "Dual Effects of Weight and Weight Gain on Breast Cancer Risk." *Journal of the American Medical Association* 278, no. 17 (1997): 1407–1411.

Hunter, D. J., et al. "Plasma Organochlorine Levels and the Risk of Breast Cancer." *New England Journal of Medicine* 337 (October 1997): 1253–1258.

Hooten, Claire. "Tai Chi: Going Through the Motions." *Consumer Reports on Health*, June 1997: 67.

Istre, O., et al. "Hormone Replacement Therapy after Transcervical Resection of the Endometrium." *American Journal of Obstetrics and Gynecology* 88 (November 1996): 767–770.

Jeffe, Donna B., et al. "Women's Reasons for Using Postmenopausal Hormone Replacement Therapy: Preventive Medicine or Therapeutic Aid?" *Menopause* 3, no. 2 (1996): 106–116.

Jurgens, Raymond W., et al. "A Comparison of Circulating Hormone Levels in Postmenopausal Women Receiving Hormone Replacement Therapy." *American Journal of Obstetrics and Gynecology* 167, no. 2 (1992): 459–460.

Kelley, Barbara Bailey. "Running on Empty." *Health*, May/June 1997: 64–68.

Kent, Howard L., M.D. "Clinical Management of Atrophic Vaginitis." *Menopause Management* 3, no. 6 (1994): 12.

Korbonen, M. O., M.D., et al. "Endometrial Biopsy Not Needed Before HRT." *American Journal of Obstetrics and Gynecology* 176 (February 1997): 377–380.

Krall, E. A., et al. "Postmenopausal Estrogen Replacement and Tooth Retention." *American Journal of Medicine* 102 (June 1997): 536–542.

Kushi, L. H., et al. "Exercise May Lower Mortality in Postmenopausal Women." *Journal of the American Medical Association* 277 (April 1997): 1287–1292.

Laan, E., et al. "Sex After Menopause." *Journal of Psychosomatic Obstetrics/Gynecology* 18 (June 1997): 126–133.

Law, M. R., et al. "A Meta-Analysis of Smoking, Bone Mineral Density, and Risk of Hip Fracture: Recognition of a Major Effect." *British Medical Journal* 315 (October 1997): 841–846.

Lindgren, R., et al. "Effects of Ginseng on Quality of Life in Postmenopausal Women." *Menopause* 4, no. 4 (1997): 245.

McNamara, R. L., et al. "Echocardiographic Identification of Cardiovascular Sources of Emboli to Guide Clinical Management of Stroke." *Annals of Internal Medicine* 127 (November 1997): 775–787.

Miller, Karen L., M.D. "Hormone Replacement Therapy in the Elderly." *Clinical Obstetrics and Gynecology* 39, no. 4 (1996): 912–932.

Myers, R. E., et al. "Analysis of Colorectal Cancer Stage among HMO Members Targeted for Screening." *Archives of Internal Medicine* 157 (September 1997): 2001–2006.

"Myths and Misperceptions about Aging and Women's Health: Initial Findings." Prepared for The National Council on the Aging by Wirthlin Worldwide. *National Council on the Aging*, November 1997: 1–10.

National Institutes of Health. "Optimal Calcium Intake." *NIH Consensus Statement* 12, no. 4 (1994).

"New Studies Find Fractures, Costs, and Prevalence Undercounted in the Past." *Osteoporosis Report* 13, no. 1 (1997): 4–5.

Nicol-Smith, L. "Causality, Menopause, and Depression: A Critical Review of the Literature." *British Medical Journal* 313 (November 1996): 1229–1232.

Nuland, Sherwin B. "Doctors and Deities." *New Republic* 217, no. 15 (October 13, 1997): 31–39.

Orlando III, Rocco, M.D. "Risk of Breast Cancer in Carriers of BRCA Gene Mutations." *New England Journal of Medicine* 337, no. 11 (1997): 787.

Ornish, Dean, M.D. "Low-Fat Diets." *New England Journal of Medicine* 338, no. 2 (1998): 127.

Paganini-Hill, Annita, Ph.D., and Victor W. Henderson, M.D. "Estrogen Replacement Therapy and Risk of Alzheimer's Disease." *Archives of Internal Medicine* 156 (October 1996): 2213–2217.

Pak, Charles Y. C., M.D., et al. "Treatment of Postmenopausal Osteoporosis with Slow-Release Sodium Fluoride." *Annals of Internal Medicine* 123, no. 6 (1996): 401–408.

Pearson, Cindy. "NCI Warns Women on Tamoxifen of Risk of Fatal Uterine Cancer Changes in Prevention Trial Consent Form Too Little, Too Late," *Network News*, March/April 1994: 4–5.

Pines, Amos, M.D., et al. "Exercise Echocardiography in Postmenopausal Hormone Users with Mild Systemic Hypertension." *American Journal of Cardiology* 78 (1996): 1385–1389.

"Postmenopausal Hormone-Replacement Therapy." *Harvard Health Publications Special Report*, January 1996: 1–38.

"Randomized Trial of Two Versus Five Years of Adjuvant Tamoxifen for Postmenopausal Early Stage Breast Cancer." *Journal of the National Cancer Institute* 88 (November 1996): 1543–1549.

Resnick, Susan M., M.D., et al. "Estrogen Replacement Therapy and Longitudinal Decline in Visual Memory." *Neurology* 49 (December 1997): 1491–1497.

Rodatra, A., et al. "Effect of Tamoxifen on Serum Estradiol Concentrations and the Development of Endometrial Pathology in Postmenopausal Women with Breast Cancer." *Menopause* 4, no. 4 (1997): 197.

Ross, D., et al. "Randomised Crossover Comparison of Skin Irritation with Two Trans-Dermal Oestradiol Patches." *British Medical Journal* 315 (August 1997): 288.

Sherwin, Barbara B. "Hormones, Mood, and Cognitive Functioning in Postmenopausal Women." *Obstetrics and Gynecology* 87, no. 2 (supplement) (1996): 205.

Shoupe, Donna, M.D. "Management of the Poor Responder to Estrogen." *Menopause Management* 5, no. 4 (1996): 20–24.

Speroff, Leon, M.D. "Compliance with Replacement Therapy." *Dialogues in Contraception* 2, no. 8 (1989): 6–8.

———. "The Comparative Effect on Bone Density, Endometrium, and Lipids of Continuous Hormones as Replacement Therapy." *Journal of the American Medical Association* 276 (November 1996): 1397–1403.

Stamper, Meir J., M.D., et al. "A Prospective Study of Postmenopausal Estrogen Therapy and Coronary Heart Disease." *New England Journal of Medicine* 313, no. 17 (1985): 1044–1049.

Stratton, J. F., et al. "Contribution of BRCA1 Mutations to Ovarian Cancer." *New England Journal of Medicine* 336 (April 1997): 1125–1130.

Swain, S. M. "Tamoxifen: The Long and Short of It." *Journal of the National Cancer Institute* 88 (November 1996): 1510–1512.

Tang, M., et al. "Effect of Oestrogen During Menopause on Risk and Age at Onset of Alzheimer's Disease." *Lancet* 348 (August 1996): 429–432.

Unger, J. B., et al. "Hysterectomy after Endometrial Ablation." *American Journal of Obstetrics and Gynecology* 175 (December 1996): 1432–1437.

Vining, Ross F., and Robynne A. McGinley. "The Measurement of Hormones in Saliva: Possibilities and Pitfalls." Proceedings of the VIIth International Congress on Hormonal Steroids (Madrid, Spain, 1986). *Pergamon Journals, Ltd.* (1987): 81–94.

Walsh, Judith, M. E., et al. "Postmenopausal Hormone Therapy: Factors Influencing Women's Decision Making." *Menopause* 4, no. 1 (1997): 39–45.

Willis, Dawn B., et al. "Estrogen Replacement Therapy and Risk of Fatal Breast Cancer in a Prospective Cohort of Postmenopausal Women in the United States." *Cancer Causes and Control* 7 (1996): 449–457.

Woolf, S. H., et al. "Preserving Scientific Debate and Patient Choice: Lessons from the Consensus Panel on Mammography Screening." *Journal of the American Medical Association* 278, no. 23 (1997): 2105–2108.

Writing Group for the PEPI Trial. "Effects of Hormone Therapy on Bone Mineral Density: Results from the Postmenopausal Estrogen/Progestin Interventions (PEPI) Trial." *Journal of the American Medical Association* 276, no. 17 (1996): 1369–1396.

Zava, David T., and Gail Duwe. "Estrogenic and Antiproliferative Properties of Genistein and Other Flavonoids in Human Breast Cancer Cells in Vitro." *Nutrition and Cancer*, 1997: 31–40.

Zhang, Yuoing, D.Sc., M.B., et al. "Bone Mass and the Risk of Breast Cancer among Postmenopausal Women." *New England Journal of Medicine* 336, no. 9 (1997): 611–617.

Self-Help Resources

Alzheimer's Disease and Related
Disorders Association
Call toll-free: 1-800-272-3900

American Association of
Acupuncture and Oriental Medicine
433 Front Street
Catasaugua, PA 18032
Call: 610-433-2448

American Cancer Society
Call toll-free: 1-800-ACS-2345

American Diabetes Association
Call toll-free: 1-800-232-3472

American Heart Association Stroke
Connection
Call toll-free: 1-800-553-6321

Cancer Information Service
(a program of the National
Cancer Institute)
Call toll-free: 1-800-4-CANCER

Endometriosis Association
Call toll-free: 1-800-992-3636

HERS Foundation
(Hysterectomy Educational
Resources and Services)
422 Bryn Mawr Avenue
Bala Cynwyd, PA 19004
Call: 610-667-7757

National Association of
Compounding Pharmacists
P.O. Box 7845
Amarillo, TX 79114
Call toll-free: 1-800-687-7694

National Eye Care Project, American
Academy of Ophthalmology
Call toll-free: 1-800-222-EYES

National Foundation for Depressive
Illness
Call toll-free: 1-800-248-4344

National Institute of Mental Health
Depression Awareness
Call toll-free: 1-800-421-4211
Panic Disorder Line
Call toll-free: 1-800-64PANIC

National Osteoporosis Foundation
2100 M Street N.W.
Suite 602, Dept. V.F.
Washington, DC 20037
Call: 202-223-2226

National Women's Health Network
Information Clearing House
514 10th St. N.W.
Washington, DC 20004
Call: 202-347-1140

North American Menopause Society
c/o University Hospitals
11100 Euclid Avenue
Cleveland, OH 44106
Call: 216-844-3334

Sexuality Information and Education
Council
80 Fifth Avenue, Suite 801
New York, NY 10011
Call: 212-819-9770

Y-Me Breast Cancer Support
Program
Call toll-free: 1-800-221-2141

Index

osteoporosis and, 27, 39, 40, 41, 43
   rheumatoid arthritis and, 55
calcitonin, 42
calorie consumption, 30, 69
Canada, 18, 66
cancer. *See also* breast cancer;
   endometrial cancer
   alcohol and, 159
   colon/rectal cancer, 32, 55–56, 58,
      144
   estrogen replacement therapy and, 32
   exercise and, 151
   hysterectomy and, 177
   lung cancer, 61, 144
   pancreatic cancer, 144
   prostate cancer, 133
   risk factors for, ix, 6
   uterine cancer, 21
   women's deaths and, 40
candy, 201–02
canola oil, 142
cantaloupe, 143, 145
cardiovascular disease
   alcohol and, 159
   coronary heart disease, 44–45, 73,
      74, 75, 76
   estrogen and, ix, 6, 58, 74–75, 87
   estrogen dosages and, 104
   estrogen replacement therapy and,
      29, 32, 44, 74, 87
   exercise and, 87, 151
   family medical history and, 72, 87
   Fempatch and, 107
   heart attacks and, 46, 61, 68, 72–
      74, 100, 124, 126
   hormone replacement therapy and,
      74, 106
   hypothyroidism and, 181
   Japanese women and, 165
   olive oil and, 143
   phytoestrogens and, 133
   raloxifene and, 124

rheumatic heart condition, 109, 142
   SERMs and, 21, 120
   soy and, 134
   tamoxifen and, 121
   vitamin E and, 142, 144
   women's deaths and, x, 40, 45, 79
Carrico, Mara, 162
carrots, 138, 143, 145
catnip, 147
cauliflower, 143, 145
Center for Risk Communications, 61–
   62
Centers for Disease Control (CDC),
   177
cereals, 195–96
cerebral amyloid, 49
chamomile, 146, 147
Chang, R. Jeffrey, 38, 109
chasteberry, 136, 146
cheese, 196–98
chemotherapy drugs, 41
cherries, 138
chicken, 143
Chinese medicine, 51, 147–48, 166
Chinese women, 166, 167
cholesterol
   antioxidants and, 144
   cardiovascular disease and, 87
   diabetes and, 76
   estrogen replacement therapy and,
      33, 73
   hormone replacement therapy and,
      74
   hypothyroidism and, 181
   soy and, 135
   tamoxifen and, 121
   tests for, 174
Chopra, Deepak, 86
climacteric, 10, 16, 54
Climara, 37, 89, 92, 94, 95, 111, 184
clitoral enlargement, 47, 48
cognitive function, ix, 22, 48, 49, 58

amenorrhea and, 9
anaerobic exercise, 151–52
breast cancer and, 79, 151
cardiovascular disease and, 87, 151
diabetes and, 75
importance of, x
Japanese women and, 165
Kegel exercises, 57–58
as lifestyle change, 150, 151–57
menopausal symptoms and, 140, 151
osteoarthritis and, 54
osteoporosis and, 27, 39, 40, 41, 43, 71, 151, 152, 157
weight-bearing exercise, 155–56
weight gain and, 30, 69, 71, 151, 158
weight training, 152, 155, 156–57, 173

family medical history. *See also* risk factors
Alzheimer's disease and, 50–51
breast cancer and, 65, 71–72
cardiovascular disease and, 72, 87
colon cancer and, 56
diabetes and, 75
estrogen decision and, 5, 32, 59, 172, 189–90
menopause and, 59
osteoporosis and, 27, 41, 72
Fareston, 122
fast foods, 208–15
fat cells, 18, 19, 29
fatigue, 33, 46–48, 104, 180–81, 181
fats (dietary), 63, 70, 78, 139, 142–43, 158–59
FDA. *See* Food and Drug Administration (FDA)
Feminine Forever (Wilson), 24, 31
Fempatch, 37, 96, 107, 111, 136, 184
fennel, 138

fiber, 56, 158
fibrinogen, 46, 100
fibroid tumors, 66–68, 177, 178
fish, 215–16
flaxseed, 133, 138
flaxseed oil, 135–36
fodder crops, 133
follicle-stimulating hormone (FSH), 4–5, 9–10, 17–18, 33, 66, 172
Food and Drug Administration (FDA)
Crinone and, 113, 117
Estratest and, 96
estrogen patches and, 37
Evista and, 43
oral micronized progesterone and, 184
Premarin and, 42, 91
Prometrium and, 113
raloxifene and, 100, 121, 125
SERMs and, 21
tamoxifen and, 122
web site of, 176
foot reflexology, 163
formication, 17
Fosamax, 42, 72
foxglove plant, 132
France, 113
free radicals, 144
frozen side dishes, 216–17
fruits, 133, 145, 158, 159, 218
FSH (follicle-stimulating hormone), 4–5, 9–10, 17–18, 33, 66, 172

gallbladder disease, 77–78, 93
garlic, 139
genistein, 133, 134
ginkgo biloba, 51, 146
Ginsana, 137
ginseng, 137, 146, 148, 166
Gladwell, Malcolm, 85–86
grains, 133, 139, 158, 159
grapefruit, 145

Greece, 142
green pepper, 139
Greer, Germaine, 187
Grodstein, Francine, 87–88
gum disorders, 56
GyneMoistrin, 99

haddock, 142
Hadza people, 165
hair, 186
Hawkes, Kristen, 165
Hayes, Helen, 187
HDL (high-density lipoprotein), 22,
    44, 45–46, 74, 97, 100, 124
Health and Human Services, U.S.
    Department of, 72
health information, 175–76, 229–36
heart, 18, 22, 123, 152, 159
Heart and Estrogen-Progestin
    Replacement Study (HERS), 74
heart attacks, 46, 61, 68, 72–74, 100,
    124, 126
heart disease. See cardiovascular
    disease
heel pains, 17
heparin, 41
herbs, 79, 136–37, 146–47, 148
herring, 142
HERS (Heart and Estrogen-Progestin
    Replacement Study), 74
high-density lipoprotein (HDL), 22,
    44, 45–46, 74, 97, 100, 124
hirsutism, 47, 48
Hook, Edward, III, 56
hops, 139
hormone replacement therapy (HRT)
    advances in, 101, 120–27
    birth control pills and, 109
    bone density tests and, 42
    breast cancer and, 64–65
    cardiovascular disease and, 74,
        106

Crinone and, 113, 117
customizing of, 85
definition of, 23
depression and, 52
estrogen dosages and, 104, 105
estrogen patches and, 95
estrogen regimens and, 115–17
Japanese women and, 165
menstrual cycles and, 76
nutrition and, 158
oral micronized progesterone and,
    184
patient-physician partnership and,
    35, 174
pregnancy and, 66
Prometrium and, 113
research studies concerning, 45–
    46
risk factors and, 35, 62
skipped pills, 184
testosterone and, 118–19
uterus and, 31–32
weight gain and, 30–31
hormones. See also specific hormones
    definition of, 19
    SERMs distinguished from, 120
Hot Flash Cookbook, The, 136
hot flashes
    Alora and, 95
    biofeedback and, 162
    description of, 27–28
    dong quai and, 136
    estrogen and, 24, 27–28
    estrogen dosages and, 103, 107
    estrogen regimens and, 118
    estrone production and, 19
    Evista and, 21
    exercise and, 151
    Fempatch and, 96
    ginseng and, 146, 166
    Japan and, 164
    Mayan Indians and, 165

as menopausal symptom, 7–8, 17, 33, 36
perimenopause and, 16
phytoestrogens and, 132, 133, 134, 135, 166
Premarin and, 104
raloxifene and, 100
Remifemin and, 136
skipped pills and, 184
surgical menopause and, 178
tamoxifen and, 121
vitamin E and, 3, 28, 109, 141–43, 144
HRT. *See* hormone replacement therapy (HRT)
Hufnagel, Vicki, 177
Hulley, Stephen B., 106
hyperthyroidism, 180
hypothalamus gland, 9–10, 15, 27
hypothyroidism, 47, 180–81
hysterectomy, 3, 11, 17, 26, 176–78

Iceland, 66
idoxifene, 125
India, 165, 167
infusion, 147
insomnia
chamomile and, 147
estrogen and, 46
estrogen dosages and, 104
exercise and, 151
as menopausal symptom, 4, 33, 36, 52
phytoestrogens and, 133
visualization and, 162
integrative medicine, 149
International Breast Cancer Screening Database Council, 66
Internet information, 175–76, 177
irritability, 36, 52
isoflavones, 133–35
Italy, 142

Jacobs Institute for Women's Health, 172
Jane Fonda's Yoga Exercise Workout, 162
Japan, 133, 134, 164–65, 166
Japanese Menopause Society, 165
Jews, 167
joint pain, 33
Jordan, V. Craig, 127

kale, 139, 142, 143
Kegel, Arnold, 57
Kegel exercises, 57–58
kelp, 143
kidney beans, 133
kidneys, 73
Kraksa, Allen, 125
K-Y Jelly, 99

Langer, Robert D., 126
LDL (low-density lipoprotein), 22, 44, 46, 51, 100, 124
Lee, Kristen, 148
lentils, 133
lettuce, 142
Levine, Mark, 145
LH (luteinizing hormone), 9–10, 18
libido, 19, 36, 47, 52–53, 96–97, 178, 185–86
licorice, 139, 146
Lie, James, 113
life expectancy, ix, 23–24, 38, 39, 58
lifestyle changes
exercise as, 150, 151–57
menopause and, 150
nutrition and, 151, 158–59
relaxation and, 161–63
stress and, 151, 159–61
lignans, 133, 135
lima beans, 133
linseed, 132

night sweats (*continued*)
  Evista and, 21
  exercise and, 151
  Fempatch and, 96
  as menopausal symptom, 7, 16, 17,
    33
  phytoestrogens and, 133, 134, 135
  Premarin and, 104
  surgical menopause and, 178
  vitamin E and, 109, 141–43
NIH (National Institutes of Health),
    25, 45, 46, 65, 71, 74, 176
*1998 Heart and Stroke Statistical
    Update* (American Heart
    Association), 45
NOF (National Osteoporosis
    Foundation), 39–40, 99, 155, 168
Nolvadex, 122
No More Hysterectomies (Hufnagel),
    177
Norlutate, 112
North American Menopause Society,
    7, 35, 168, 173, 192
Northrup, Christiane, 35
Notelovitz, Morris, 97, 98
Nurses' Health Study, 44, 46, 74, 87–
    88, 151
nutrition
  breast cancer and, 79
  calcium and, 33, 70, 158, 193–226
  cardiovascular disease and, 87
  high-fat diets and, 63, 78
  Japanese women and, 165
  lifestyle changes and, 151, 158–59
  nutritional supplements, 140
  phytoestrogens and, 133, 136
  reduced-fat diets and, 70, 158–59
  weight gain and, 70–71, 158
nuts, 221

oats, 139
Ogen, 18–19, 111

olive oil, 139, 142, 143
*150 Most-Asked Questions About
    Menopause* (Jacobowitz), 6
*150 Most-Asked Questions About
    Midlife Sex, Love, and Intimacy*
    (Jacobowitz), 6
*150 Most-Asked Questions About
    Osteoporosis* (Jacobowitz), 6
onions, 139
OPAL (Osteoporosis Prevention and
    Artery Effects of Tibolone), 126
oral estrogens, 88, 90, 111
oral micronized progesterone, 45, 46–
    47, 52, 106, 113, 117, 184–85
oranges, 145
Ortho, 111
Ortho-Est, 88, 111
osteoarthritis, 32, 54–55, 58, 142
osteoblasts, 43
osteoporosis. *See also* bone
  breast cancer and, 88
  Estratab and, 98
  estrogen and, ix, 6, 22, 39–40, 58,
    74
  estrogen dosages and, 102, 103, 104
  estrogen replacement therapy and,
    29, 32
  exercise and, 27, 39, 40, 41, 43,
    151, 152, 157
  Fempatch and, 107
  Japanese women and, 165
  osteoarthritis compared to, 54
  prevention of, 27
  raloxifene and, 21, 100, 124–25
  research studies and, 42, 43, 100,
    126–27
  as risk factor, x
  SERMs and, 100
  soy and, 134
  surgical menopause and, 97
  teeth and, 56
  Women's Health Initiative and, 75

phytosterol creams, 137
phytosterols, 146–47
Pike, Malcolm, 117
pituitary gland, 9–10, 15
Pizzorno, Joseph, 51
plant estrogens. *See* phytoestrogens
PMS, 76, 105–06, 136
polyunsaturated oils, 142
pomegranate, 139
Postmenopausal Estrogen-Progestin
    Intervention (PEPI), 45–46, 72
postmenopausal women
  alendronate and, 43
  breast cancer and, 64
  estrogen needs of, 29, 37
  estrone production and, 17, 18
  exercise and, 151
  Fareston and, 122
  osteoporosis and, 39, 127
  phytoestrogens and, 132
  pregnancy and, 66
  SERMs and, 124, 126
  status of, 165, 167, 168, 187
Power Surge, 176
pregnancy
  breast cancer and, 63
  estriol production and, 17, 18
  estrogen replacement therapy and,
    28, 66
  and menstrual cycles, 9, 10, 15
  progesterone production and, 20
Premarin
  Alora and, 95
  Alzheimer's disease and, 50–51
  description of, 90–91
  dosages of, 90, 102–05, 111
  early use of, 24
  effectiveness of, 21, 37, 83
  gallbladder disease and, 77
  as natural estrogen, 89
  as oral estrogen, 88
  osteoporosis and, 42

PEPI trial and, 45
  as vaginal cream, 91, 112
premenstrual syndrome, 76, 105–06,
    136
Premphase, 77, 91, 112, 184
Prempro, 77, 91, 106, 112, 184
progesterone
  changes in production of, 16, 17
  educational materials on, 175
  functions of, 9–10, 19–20
  hormone replacement therapy and,
    23, 52
  oral micronized progesterone, 45, 46–
    47, 52, 106, 113, 117, 184–85
  product choices of, 112
  replacement of, 11
  surgical menopause and, 26, 177
progesterone challenge test, 33
progestin
  endometrial cancer and, 25, 60
  estrogen patches and, 92, 95
  hormone replacement therapy and,
    23, 31–32, 37, 116
  menstrual cycles and, 76
  mental tonic effect and, 46–47, 105–
    06
  PEPI trials and, 45–46
  Prempro and, 91
  product choices of, 112
prolapse, 177
Promensil, 134
Prometrium, 113
prostate cancer, 133
protein, 41, 140, 142, 158, 218
Provera, 45, 105–06, 112, 113
pulmonary emboli, 68
pumpkin, 143
pyorrhea, 56
pyridoxine, 143

qi gong, 163
Quigley, Ted, 119

thrombophlebitis, 68
thyroid function, 33
thyroid gland, 175, 180–81
thyroid medication, 41
thyroid stimulating hormone assay
    (TSH), 180–81
tibolone, 126
Timmons, M. Chrystie, 97
tincture, 147
Today's Therapeutic Trends 1996,
    103
tofu, 135
tomato, 143
Tonganese women, 167
transdermal therapy, 37, 88–89. *See
    also* estrogen patches
Tri-estrogen, 89
triglyceride levels, 33, 73, 76, 100, 124
TSH (thyroid stimulating hormone
    assay), 180–81
tuna, 143

U.S. Government web site, 176
urinary incontinence, ix, x, 56–58, 98,
    108
urinary tract infections (UTIs), 56–57
urogenital atrophy, 98
uterine cancer, 21
uterus
    continuous combined therapy and,
        76, 91
    Crinone and, 113
    droloxifene and, 125
    Estring and, 108
    estrogen and, 18, 60
    estrogen patches and, 92, 95
    estrogen regimens and, 115–17
    hormone replacement therapy and,
        23, 31–32, 37, 115–17
    progesterone and, 46
    progestin and, 25, 95

SERMs and, 100, 120, 121, 122,
    123, 124
surgical menopause and, 26, 177
uterine fibroid tumors, 66–68, 177,
    178
UTIs (urinary tract infections), 56–57

vaginal atrophy, 141
vaginal cream, 72–73, 91, 98–99, 108,
    111–12
vaginal dryness
    estrogen and, 24
    estrogen dosages and, 103
    estrogen replacement therapy and,
        52
    Evista and, 21
    Fempatch and, 107
    as menopausal symptom, 33, 36
    phytoestrogens and, 133
    Premarin and, 105
    vitamin E and, 141, 144
vaginal lubricants, 99
vaginal ultrasound, 33
valerian root, 147
Valium, 4
vegetables, 133, 145, 158, 159, 224–
    26
visualization, 79, 162
vitamin A, 143, 144
vitamin B_6, 143
vitamin C, 144, 145
vitamin E, 3, 28, 109, 134, 141–43,
    144
vitamins
    dosage of, 148
    fiber and, 158
    menopausal symptoms and, 3, 28,
        79, 109, 134, 140–43, 144
    multivitamins, 145–46
Vivelle 37, 92, 95–96, 107, 111
voice deepening, 47, 48

About the Author

Ruth S. Jacobowitz is an award-winning medical writer, a dynamic lecturer, a columnist, and a former vice president of a large university-affiliated teaching hospital in Cleveland, Ohio. This is her fifth book on the subject of women's midlife health, a subject that she says has become her permanent "beat." The author of *150 Most-Asked Questions About Menopause; 150 Most-Asked Questions About Osteoporosis;* and *150 Most-Asked Questions About Midlife Sex, Love, and Intimacy,* she is also co-author, with Wulf H. Utian, M.D., of *Managing Your Menopause.*

Ruth Jacobowitz's engaging and informative lectures have taken her all over the world, where with warmth, wit, and wisdom she educates women about how they age and empowers them to take charge of their health. She was the only lay speaker invited to the World Congress on Fertility and Sterility in Montpelier, France, to speak to physicians about "Women's Perspectives on HRT." She has been featured on *48 Hours, Today, CBS This Morning, Donahue, Leeza, Marilu, America's Talking,* Food Television Network, *Morning Exchange, Company, Good Company,* and *People Are Talking,* as well as on television shows in many cities, on the news, and in major newspapers and magazines, and on *National Public Radio* and local radio shows throughout North America.

Listed in *Who's Who in the World* and *Who's Who in American Women,* Ruth Jacobowitz is a member of the National

Council on Women's Health, a trustee of the Doris A. Howell Foundation for Women's Health Research, a founding member of the North American Menopause Society, a member of the International Menopause Society, and a former Midwest chair of the Association of American Medical Colleges Group on Public Affairs.

Ruth Jacobowitz and her husband, Paul, have been married for more than forty years. They live in La Jolla, California, and are the parents of three married daughters and the grandparents of eight, four girls and four boys.